Why Should We Care?

Edited by

Donald Evans

Centre for the Study of Philosophy and Health Care University College Swansea

M

MACMILLAN
PRESS
Scientific & Medical

First published 1990

Published by
THE MACMILLAN PRESS LTD
Houndmills, Basingstoke, Hampshire RG21 2XS
and London
Companies and representatives
throughout the world

Printed in Hong Kong

British Library Cataloguing in Publication Data
Why should we care? – (Professional studies in health care ethics).
1. Health services. Ethical aspects
I. Evans, Donald, *1939–* II. Series
174'.2
ISBN 0–333–51562–5
ISBN 0–333–51563–3 pbk

WHY SHOULD WE CARE?

PROFESSIONAL STUDIES IN HEALTH-CARE ETHICS

Much that has been written about ethical problems in health care has been authored by philosophers and lawyers. By contrast this series provides a platform for practitioners to address their colleagues on these important issues, having benefited from training in philosophical reflection. The volumes in the series will be of interest to professional health carers and the general public alike as the issues discussed are frequently presented for general attention by the media.

Contents

Preface

There is an inevitable moral dimension to health-care provision. This collection of essays demonstrates that inevitability and begins to explore the complexity of this dimension. The issues are of public concern, and all concerned with health care, whether as providers or consumers, should reflect on them. This volume will engage practitioners and members of the general public in the growing debate.

The essays are written by a variety of people who have either taught or studied at the Swansea Centre for Philosophy and Health Care. The authors tackle central ethical questions arising in various specialties and provide a welcome voice on these matters from within health-care practice.

Thanks are due to the many colleagues of the authors at The Centre, and to the faculty of the Centre, who have provided the stimulation of multi-disciplinary discussion and the guidance in reflection respectively, which together have produced the confidence required to commit thoughts to paper on these issues of moment.

Notes on the Contributors

Peter Beck is a Consultant Physician for South Glamorgan Health Authority and Hon. Secretary of the Ethics Committee in Medicine of The Royal College of Physicians.

Richard Bentall is a Lecturer at the Department of Clinical Psychology, University of Liverpool.

Donald Evans is Director of The Centre for Philosophy and Health Care, University College Swansea.

Naomi Gilchrist is a Lecturer in Social Care, at Basford Hall College of Further Education.

Paul Goulden is a Consultant Anaesthetist with the Yorkshire Regional Health Authority.

Alan Hawley is a Specialist in Occupational Medicine with the British Army.

Eve MacGregor is a Health Visitor currently raising a young family.

David Moore is Divisional Head, Dorset & Salisbury College of Midwifery & Nursing.

Patrick Nash is a Senior Lecturer in Nursing Studies, Swansea College of Higher Education.

Sylvia Parker is a Nursing Officer with the Mid-Glamorgan Area Health Authority.

Michael Saunders is a Consultant Neurologist with the Northern Regional Health Authority.

Denise Skiffington is a GP in Bowden, South Australia.

1 Why Should We Care?

Donald Evans

The question 'Why should we care?', which is commonly used to disclaim moral responsibility, has a hollow ring when applied to the role of professional health carers. There is no obligation on anyone to become a doctor, nurse, pharmacist, health visitor or related health-care professional. Nevertheless once such a role is adopted, moral responsibilities automatically come as part of the package. But so, it may be argued, do they come when one adopts the role of mechanic, tailor, or airline pilot. It is of course true that to become involved in any employee/employer, producer/consumer, professional/client relationship brings with it moral duties and corresponding rights. Indeed in the case of the motor mechanic and perhaps even more obviously in that of the airline pilot the safety and health of the customer is a matter of considerable importance. This is true insofar as prevention of harm due to negligence, overwork or some such consideration must play a major role in the determination of whether one is a good mechanic or pilot.

But here the similarities end. If I am to be a good doctor or nurse I must not merely be a loyal employee and a careful, technically skilled practitioner. There is something in the very nature of the work I am to do and the subsequent relationship with those who are the subject matter of my work which has a moral dimension. This dimension may itself make the work more problematic. It will also make it more personally demanding. To ignore this dimension of health-care provision and practice will not simply make one an inefficient manager or practitioner. It will render one morally culpable and a positive danger.

Perhaps health carers are not unique in this regard. That will depend partly on how widely one draws the limits of the concept of health. No doubt a case could be made for such a dimension attaching to the role of educators and politicians for example. It is not the purpose of this collection of essays to establish uniqueness in this sense. It is its purpose, however, to begin to draw out the pervasive and thoroughgoing role of values in health-care practice and provision.

Careful attempts to identify and analyse the business of values in medicine and health care generally have only relatively recently begun in earnest. This is not to say that practitioners by and large have been neglectful of the moral aspects of their practice until now. No doubt some have. It would be surprising if that were not so. However, for various reasons, even those who have been highly sensitive to these matters find themselves in need of the kind of help recent analysis has begun to provide.

What has changed to make the health carer so anxious about these questions? There are numbers of considerations that have conspired to generate the current intensity of interest in medical ethics and health-care ethics generally.

First, litigation against practitioners has concentrated the minds of health professionals on the question of what they ought to do in various situations. Whilst this concern is not essentially moral in that it is largely about what it is safe for the practitioner to do to protect his interests if challenged in the courts, it is not unconnected with moral propriety. It is true that legal and ethical propriety do not always coincide. However they are not totally unrelated. This relation is demonstrated in the process of legislation which is often stimulated by the moral demand to regulate some practice or other. In medical research such controls have been sought from time to time. The example in Great Britain of the setting-up of a government commission chaired by Baroness Warnock, a philosopher, to advise on the framing of legislation involving the control of research on human embryos and the use of various techniques in infertility treatment is a case in point. Similarly there are calls for control in research in genetic engineering in humans. Whilst litigation has played a major role in stimulating interest in medical ethics in the USA, its influence has been less marked, though not absent, in Europe. Currently the row about the procurement of human organs for transplantation has involved a possible court case and sent ethics committees back to their drawing boards to examine the issues.

Second, the move towards greater freedom of information and openness in Western societies has led to a sharper awareness of individual rights. The placing of the Data Protection Act on the Statute Book in Great Britain has raised the question of to whom the information held about a patient belongs, with consequent problems about confidentiality and a challenge to the traditional medical paternalism. This has brought the question of informed consent out in bolder relief than ever. It is evidence of a remarkable shift in moral priorities in health-care practice from the principle of beneficence to that of the autonomy of the individual.

Third, and maybe most dramatically, the explosion of high tech medicine and drug therapies has engaged the attention of practitioners and public alike to moral issues in health care. Doctors now have the power to do things which less than a generation ago seemed unthinkable. Human life can be generated in vitro, rogue genes can be screened in very early stages of pregnancy, vital organs can be transplanted from one human being to another, machines can perform the functions of heart, lungs and kidneys so that life can be artificially prolonged, indefinitely in some cases, and so on. Each of these new capabilities brings with it new choices and demands. Because something can be done does it follow that it should be done? And if it should be done in one case should it be done in another? And if not, how shall we know the difference? Because the practitioner has the power to perform such feats should he also carry the responsibility of deciding whether or not he should so act?

Doctors currently have to bear this moral burden and many find it a lonely and extremely demanding role. Their training as clinicians has not prepared them for identifying and weighing up the relevant pros and cons. It seems that they are expected to play the role of God without the endowment of divine wisdom. It is therefore no surprise that many seek support and assistance.

The fourth major stimulus to interest in health-care ethics is the scarcity of resources in health care. There is hardly a week goes by in the United Kingdom when some crisis in the Health Service does not arise which is directly attributable to shortage of resources. Talk of efficiency measures often masks lack of funding; quality of care takes second place to achievement of financial targets; staff are overstretched; waiting lists grow longer; preferred therapies are threatened because of the cost of the best medicines; centralisation of services further erodes just distribution of health-care provision. And on and on it goes. In this situation discussion of what ought to be provided and on what basis, professional standards of care and accountability, measurement of quality of care, and numerous other issues has flourished. These are exciting days for the study of the ethics of health care. Awareness of such problems and the determination on the part of health carers to equip themselves to grapple with them in reflection as well as practice cannot but be good for the provision of health care.

Finally the emergence of the international health problem of AIDS has drawn members of all sections of the professions and public at large into the discussion of medico-moral questions. Whilst it presents no new ethical issues it certainly brings old issues like confidentiality, compulsory screening and care, assisted death and various other problems into the public arena. But to whom can the professionals turn for help in the analysis of these perplexing issues? As a matter of fact they have turned in growing numbers to the philosopher. This has been somewhat of a shock to some members of the medical establishment and indeed to the general public. Philosophers have traditionally, or at least for a long time, occupied the penthouse of the ivory tower of Academe. Divorced from the real problems faced by ordinary mortals they have been preoccupied with questions such as 'Is "God" a proper name?', 'How can I know who I am?', 'Is time real?', and so on. If we consider the nature of some of the skills the philosopher has to bring to the problems with which we are now concerned, we may see some wisdom in enlisting his aid. But first a word about the natural defensiveness felt by health-care professionals at the approach of the philosopher.

It is to be expected that any professional group will feel threatened by another group which appears to tell it how it should conduct its affairs. This is especially so when such advice is issued from the detached and comfortable vantage point of the armchair and not from a position of engagement in the consulting room, on the ward or in the intensive care unit. A commonplace rejoinder to the philosopher who dares to engage in discussion of medical ethical issues with a clinician is: 'Have you ever had clinical responsibility for a patient?' Understandably so. It is all too easy to make decisions for others when they cost one nothing at all. But care is needed lest what the philosopher may have to offer which is of value is not discounted in haste and repented of at leisure. If there are distinctive skills which the philosopher can bring to the aid of the professional health carer may they be welcomed for what they are and not rejected because of whence they come.

Philosophers have a certain kind of interest in the activities of the artist, the artisan, the scientist, the politician and the worshipper. This may suggest, at first blush, that they are busybodies intruding into areas where they have no proper business. Their interest in medical ethics has been construed in just this light:

> Having left its house untended while taking a long technological holiday, the medical profession should not be altogether surprised on returning home to find a number of squatters in occupation . . . mainly comprising a group of moral philosophers seeking work . . . medicine as a profession can and should put its own ethical house in order . . . in the confidence that overall we are better educated, better informed, and better motivated, in matters to do with medical practice and its organisation, than those who are bidding to take over parts of our work.[1]

However, philosophers have a legitimate interest in questions of health-care practice. To appreciate this suspicion of philosophical analysis and to eliminate it from the mind of the reader of this collection of essays, and of other collections in this Series, let us briefly review two levels of analysis at which the philosopher operates. They illustrate the usefulness of his skills to the professional health carer who wishes to confront the problems we have earlier marked out as calling for attention.

First, the philosopher is trained to unravel conceptual confusions which may occur in areas specific to certain disciplines or activities. Second, he is interested in clarifying what is involved in whole ways of talking and thinking. Examples of the first would be found in an examination of questions such as: 'When does human life begin?', 'Is mental illness really illness?', 'Is health simply the absence of disease?' Examples of the second would be constituted by an examination of the nature of moral judgements.

It is not difficult to see that analyses of some of the questions at the first level could make a difference to the activities of the practitioner. The dispute between psychiatry and so called anti-psychiatry[2] is an example of philosophical dispute at this level which is presently far from being resolved. The Szasz position places considerable question marks over the manner in which many 'psychiatric patients' are currently treated. If it is not the case that psychiatrically disturbed people have a disease of the mind, then they should not be compulsorily detained for treatment and neither should they be absolved from responsibility for their actions over which they cannot properly be said to lack control. Now it may well be that practitioners committed to a medical model of mental illness feel threatened by the kind of analysis called for in the dispute with anti-psychiatrists. Nevertheless, philosophical analysis is a quest for clarity about the identity of mental illness and is not designed to bolster or undermine accepted practice. If, as a result of such analysis, doubt is thrown on one or other mode of handling psychiatric cases then such doubt should, in the name of good health care, be welcomed and taken seriously.

The second level of analysis is explicitly related to the moral dimension of health-care practice and provision. It is here that opposition to the philosopher's activities has been most pointed. This is in part due to a division within philosophy between those who believe that philosophy is capable of answering substantive moral questions and those who believe that its business is simply to clarify. No-one enjoys moral lectures, especially from strangers. When some of the way out recommendations from moral philosophers[3] fall upon the ears of health carers they recoil and understandably so, but so do many philosophers. Nevertheless some unravelling of the relevant considerations which go to make up a moral problem cannot but assist the practitioner grappling with the problems to make some headway. Not that this will make health-care practice easier. The result may be quite the reverse. Reflection may bring out just how difficult and serious many decisions are, and this could come as a surprise. Practice may consequently be more difficult but it could hardly be the poorer. To resist such analysis, to play the role of the proverbial ostrich in matters of morality in health care must be a reaction deprecated by all responsible practitioners.

The essays which follow have been collected to illustrate both levels of analysis outlined above. Some refer to general questions of the nature of moral action and decision making in health-care practice. Others tackle specific conceptual issues which have considerable bearing on the question of what ought or ought not to be done. They are almost all authored by health-care professionals who have benefited from philosophical training and who are thus able to bring the hard edge of experience to bear upon philosophical reflection.

Alan Hawley, in 'Morality and Patient Care', points out the inevitability of the moral dimension in health-care practice. It is argued that the relation between the practitioner and the patient invokes a multi-layered moral context for practice. It is not a question of adding a moral gloss to the provision of health care. By its nature such provision embodies moral demands and to ignore them is to degrade the activity. Health-care cannot of itself be a morally neutral business.

Moral values inevitably enter health-care practice in another way, namely, at the level of diagnosis. Diagnosis itself may often be seen as a form of moral intervention. The case is trenchantly argued by Richard Bentall in 'Values in Diagnosis', where he concentrates on the diagnoses of psychiatric disorders. How far does the value content of diagnosis stretch? Illness and disease point out negatively valued conditions. But is the direction of this relation a clear one? Might not many negatively valued conditions be classified as diseases simply as an indication of the value placed on them by a given culture? The question is provocative. Bentall suggests an interesting extension of such evaluation in diagnosis beyond psychiatry, causing us to reflect on the much vaunted objective character of medical science. Insofar as the thesis holds we cannot help but exhibit value preferences in health-care practice.

To call attention to the presence of moral values in health care is not the end of the story for the professional carer. Alertness to these values will often present the carer with anxieties otherwise avoided. Morality is not a tidy whole and its multiple demands may conflict and produce dilemmas. Michael Saunders' essay 'Moral Dilemmas in Health Care' illustrates and examines the kind of perplexity which is produced by such conflicts. He explores possible routes of escape from such situations, but doubts their adequacy. Some moral burdens are harder to bear than others; perhaps the hardest are those that demand that something be done when all the alternatives are dreadful. His analysis may console colleagues who have laboured under this particular load whilst not in any way absolving them from responsibility for deeds done. To know that there need not be a solution to every moral problem, a route out of every apparent impasse, may constitute at once a greater understanding of morality and sustenance to carers struggling with dilemmas or memories of choices made which are hard to live with.

As surely as conflicts may arise between moral demands made on the individual carer, conflicts may arise between the views of different carers. Taking morality seriously will bring one, from time to time, into disagreement with others. Such disagreements may need to be resolved before care can continue to be provided. How can we set about resolving such differences, if we can resolve them at all? Eve MacGregor examines a popular method of resolution in 'Moral Disputes in Health Care'. A weighing up of the consequences of alternative actions, especially in terms of the sum total of happiness or welfare produced, seems to hold out great promise. Consequences certainly cannot be disregarded but do they alone win the day?

Few disputes have raised the temperature as high as that over the status of the human foetus. It is a central issue in discussion of abortion, embryo research, use of foetal tissue for research and transplant purposes, genetic engineering, genetic screening, surrogacy and so on. Naomi Gilchrist explores the adequacy of consequentialist arguments to establish certain claims about the foetus in 'The Status of the Foetus'. In the process she raises fundamental questions about the duty to care. But can philosophy tell us ultimately how we should treat the foetus? Or indeed for that matter how we should treat a viable but handicapped neonate? Sylvia Parker examines the kind of illumination which may be gained from philosophical reflection about the nature of such a discussion. 'Should my Baby Live?' shows clearly that reflection may make decisions more difficult but only because it makes the issues about which decisions are to be made clearer. If the situations are more complex and morally demanding than we had at first realised we do better to care enough to reflect, so that the decision will be responsible and informed, though albeit more painful.

To extend proper care to an individual may make great demands on us to reflect. But so may the question of those to whom we should extend care. Given that there are inevitable limits on resources and widespread demand for care, how can we care adequately? David Moore, in 'The Limits of Health Care', explores the various economic models employed to allocate scarce resources. He identifies the consequentialist rationale that underpins them. He raises the problem of the identity and aggregation of benefits and argues that they are shot through with values though they are paraded as being value-free. Measurement of quality of life has its own problems but the employment of such a measure to determine who shall be cared for raises serious questions about the value of a life.

It is precisely this question which is taken up by Denise Skiffington in 'Experiments on People and Animals'. She is concerned with issues that arise in medical research. She asks whether it is those features of human beings that differentiate them from animals which increase their moral significance. She rejects purposiveness, rationality, and so on, as being constitutive of the value of a life though she stresses the importance of autonomy. That theme is further developed by Paul Goulden in his review of the ethical issues raised by drug development, and it becomes the central theme of Peter Beck's essay on 'Informed Consent'.

The case of 'informed consent' has been championed above any other in medical ethics. It is tied to the concept of competence.

It is precisely this facility to make autonomous choices which is compromised in mental illness. Patrick Nash, in 'Autonomy, Competence and Mental Disorders' brings out the necessity of determining competence to consent in giving proper care to the mentally disordered. Competence is not a seamless whole and one needs to guard against the 'Catch 22' position in which patients maybe trapped. Consent is sought (apparently on the presumption of competence). If it is given then competence is not questioned and treatment goes ahead. If it is refused this is taken to be a criterion of incompetence and the treatment goes ahead anyway. It may be felt that the informal patient stands in great risk of being treated with less respect than is proper because of the nature of the condition to be treated.

It is but a small step to compulsory care. Here we meet, in psychiatric medicine, a firm answer to our question 'Why should we care?', but is it an unambiguous answer? The state has decreed that in certain cases of psychiatric disorder, care should be given without consent. Richard Bentall in 'The Abuse of Psychiatry' presents a powerful case for handling such provisions with extreme sensitivity. Whose interests are served by compulsory detention and treatment? Are we sure that western practice is free of those abuses identified in psychiatry elsewhere? Are our grounds for compulsory care really based in a concern to care for the disordered person?

The following essays are not presented as answers to any specific questions in health-care ethics. They constitute a response to the question 'Why should we care?' and, it is hoped, they show what is wrong with asking the question.

Notes

1. John A. Davis. 'Whose life is it anyway?', *British Medical Journal* (April 1986) vol. 292, p. 1128.
2. See especially Thomas Szasz, *The Myth of Mental Illness* (New York: Hoeber-Harper, 1961).
3. See, for example, the proposal to use healthy human beings as involuntary banks of donor organs in John Harris, *Violence and Responsibility* (London: Routledge, Kegan Paul, 1980); and 'The Survival Lottery', *Philosophy* (1975) vol. 50, pp. 81–7.

2 Morality and Patient Care

Alan Hawley

The provision of health care in the United Kingdom is a concept which has largely been taken for granted since the introduction of the National Health Service. In recent years, with a growing mismatch between demand and resources, many have come to question the methods by which health care is dispensed. As ever, when available resources fail to meet demand, hard choices are necessary. The crucial question is: on what criteria should those options be chosen? Faced with this problem many would feel that moral aspects have to play a part in any equation. The majority would probably accept that proposition. Nevertheless, it remains to be demonstrated why moral concerns do and should affect the provision of health care.

Happily for most people, the provision of health care merely involves an occasional visit to the family doctor. At this individual level there are a number of tacitly accepted conventions. For instance, the maintenance of confidentiality and truth-telling are expected. Other principles that may well be anticipated include consent before any further referral or investigations are done and a respect by the doctor for the autonomy of the patient. Normally these principles are never enunciated by either party but are merely assumed. Without this arrangement it becomes very difficult for any consultation to operate. The requirement for the patient to be able to trust the medical practitioner is paramount. This is particularly true in any serious or chronic condition.

Since illness or disability makes people more vulnerable both physically and emotionally, the necessity of trust becomes crucial. This places the doctor in both a privileged and responsible position. He is privileged in being able to help and assist another fellow human but is burdened by the responsibility that flows from this. In practical terms any decisions that may be made both therapeutic and managerial, will have some effect upon the patient's life. This may be a minor result such as abstention from alcohol involved in some therapeutic regimes, or a major change in lifestyle as in recommendation for withdrawal of driving licence in certain epileptics.

Any situation where a person in a position of trust makes decisions affecting another more vulnerable individual, has a moral aspect. It is inevitable that occupations requiring involvement, often intimate, in others' lives will also involve moral concerns. The nature of these concerns may differ but they remain essentially moral. This fits the popular perception of a doctor. He is seen as a person who places the interest of his patients before self. However imperfect this model, it is one that provides both comfort and reassurance to most potential and actual patients.[1]

The presence of moral perspectives in health care is brought into sharp focus when a conflict occurs between different principles. This may be a conflict essentially confined to one partner in a consultation. Such a situation arises when the consequences of telling the whole truth to a patient is judged by the doctor as potentially psychologically damaging. This decision to withhold important details cuts across the principle of respect for patients' autonomy. The difficulty lies in resolving the dilemma. Even compromising on the details of the condition will not tackle the core of the problem. Fundamentally, the two moral principles are irreconcilable on occasions. It is at these times that the consequences of the ultimate decision become the dominant factor. The final working out of the problem will frequently be achieved by consideration of the relative results of both courses. It is by the very process of recognition and resolution of a dilemma that the moral nature of the doctor–patient consultation is demonstrated.

This problem of moral conflict is particularly difficult when the difference exists between doctor and patient. Whilst a moral difficulty perceived by a doctor in his choice of treatments is not infrequent, it is often resolved without direct patient input. Many people would be unaware of any ethical problem faced by their medical practitioner. However, some issues show up differences in moral outlook between the parties in a consultation. Probably the most obvious example is abortion. It is clearly impossible to reconcile a practitioner's belief in the absolute wrongness of abortion with a patient's wish to have her pregnancy terminated. This may have far reaching consequences. Not only can it radically affect the solution of that particular problem, but if mutual trust and respect are damaged, the whole future relationship between the two may be undermined. In this specific example, the presence of a conscientious objection clause in the Abortion Act allows both parties to circumvent the problem. The Abortion Act is further evidence of the moral contract which exists between doctor and patient, since recognition of a right to conscientious abstention is an implicit acceptance of a moral dimension.

Important though the exchange is between the individual players in a consultation, they are working in a moral climate set by society. In the above example, society, through parliamentary action, has set definitions and ground rules for abortion by use of the Abortion Act. The statute book is one way of establishing an ethical milieu. However, there is also the climate of opinion which may be at variance with the laws of the land. This may in some way reflect a popular perception of natural justice and the norms of civilised behaviour. The importance of this phenomenon is that it helps formulate the ground rules and provides the background for the practice of medicine.[2]

This is of fundamental significance when the next level of health-care provision is examined. Having explored the ethical nature of the individual consultation, it now becomes necessary to review the problem of resource allocation. Whilst there would be general agreement on the moral nature at the level of the consulting room, the problem becomes more convoluted at the higher level.

The allocation of resources is a function of government. In democratic countries the right and legitimacy to do this derives from the ballot box and through that the expression of the electorate's will. There is an obvious political factor in deciding how the national cake will be divided up. One would expect differences in emphasis between different political parties. Also, there is a fundamental and integral relationship between a moral outlook and a political view. Hence, the political factor is itself a mixture of different elements. Equally, economic factors will have to be weighed in the balance. The record of national wealth generation will be a major deciding factor in the ultimate apportioning of resources. No responsible government will risk financial catastrophe by over ambitious plans. There has to be at least an approximate marrying up of assets to plans.

However, not many societies find themselves with the luxury of being able to afford everything. At that point choices have to be made. An important factor in these choices will be moral outlook. Thus, some would choose to spend more on social schedules such as education, health and social security. Others regard the maintenance of national sovereignty and identity as paramount and support more resources being diverted to defence and industrial development. Indeed, there is an argument that spending on health care does not improve the general well being of the population. It is social change and improved standard of living that achieves this. Certainly, examples exist of improvement in social conditions which have led to the controlling of diseases. The reduction in prevalence of tuberculosis in the United Kingdom during this century was due largely to an amelioration in housing standards and better nutrition.[3] On the other hand, there are other examples of applied health-care reducing hazards. For example, the elimination of smallpox was achieved by a policy of vaccination.

This problem of the efficacy of treatment presents further difficulties in resource allocation. Having decided the total amount to be spent on health services, it then requires the budget to be apportioned between the competing medical demands. Thus preventive schemes and curative regimes have to be balanced. Funding does not exist for all.

One moral basis for any overall health cover is that of utilitarianism. Put boldly and simply this requires that the greatest good be achieved for the greatest number.[4] The concept may appear to resolve many ethical problems. It is certainly the principle that is followed by the Army Medical Services in war. However, the demands of peacetime are rather more complex. The very attraction of utilitarianism, its essential simplicity, does not meet the myriad of difficulties faced by an increasing demand in society.

Utilitarians would argue that preventive schemes are usually preferable to curative. They are definitely more desirable than expensive care for the incurably and terminally ill. To be consistent, a utilitarian outlook would advocate palliative and supportive treatment for these groups. Some might even consider euthanasia in one way or another. Such a view whilst having the merit of being logically consistent seems to be lacking in compassion and sinister in its implications.

It is this aspect of sympathy and consideration for the most unfortunate, which comprises the concept of justice. This is an important moral factor. It is in the popular conscience and forms an indispensable component of the ethical medium. To many people it is an often unstated but powerful feeling. The belief in fairness of care and treatment is a crucial element in this. Indeed, one of the most reviled aspects of Nazi society was their flaunting of this particular tenet. By their execution and ill treatment of the physically and mentally disabled, the Nazis outraged popular democratic opinion. Arguably, the National Socialist Party could have asserted that they were following the logical moral outlook of utilitarianism. This would suggest that even the Nazis believed they had a moral basis for action. Importantly, it also shows the significance of natural justice to popular democratic societies. The maintenance of this perceived justice is a deeply ingrained element of this ethical outlook.

The evaluation of consequences in different choices of health care is also important in formulating a policy. This consideration of the results can emphasise the moral basis of the caring system. It also means that some sort of objective calculation has to be attempted. Comparing the relative merits of a preventive scheme against a clinical treatment is an invidious and difficult uncertainty. Generally, whilst the results of preventive medicine may be to reduce the incidence of a condition, they remain largely statistical and hence theoretical gains. However, the immediacy of the requirement for a transplant or critical care is much more tangible. This very difference works in favour of the curative options. To deny someone the required treatment without which they might die, denies the principle of natural justice. In recent months the controversy over shortages of beds in paediatric intensive therapy units has graphically illustrated this point. The net effect of this tendency is to promote the development of treatment at the expense of preventive policies. The inevitable personalisation of the question into a dilemma for an individual lends poignancy to the situation. Against this, prophylactic options must depend upon statistical evidence.

Nevertheless, within the curative options there remains the difficulty in selection. Modern medicine is a most expensive business. The cost rises at higher than the rate of inflation, primarily driven by the expense of new technologies. This means that priorities have to be allocated. Here the choices are much more difficult. Frequently, there is a plethora of moral principles employed. Thus, a hybrid utilitarianism may be born. Generally, utilitarian criteria will be employed tempered by concern for natural justice. The cynical might call this a policy of crisis management. Since it is fundamentally reactive, there may be some truth in this. The hybrid option relies upon policies being employed for the greater good but with additional resources being diverted into single deserving projects. Usually, these will become obvious where a crisis has arisen. To this extent the option does indeed become one of studied crisis management.

Another option which seems to be favoured currently in the United Kingdom and the USA is for the state to undertake certain minimum levels of care. Normally these will include provision for the acutely critical ill, the chronically ill and those who are economically disadvantaged. Other than these areas it becomes the responsibility of the individual to provide for his own care. The moral principle is one of sharing the growing burden of health funding.[5] This, it is argued, releases resources for other policies. Clearly, the danger with this policy is one of tiering in health care. The risk exists that a two tier system will evolve. Whatever the arguments, there is an undoubted moral aspect to both sides. That is the crucial fact.

Avoiding this option many countries adopt a form of rotational financing. Using this policy, which may actually be inadvertent, over a period of some years a cyclical pattern in funding can be identified. Each health requirement is given priority in turn. This means that over the whole cycle all requirements will have been both met and underfunded. It is a variation of the hybrid utilitarian approach.

Once the hard choices about overall resource allocation have been made, the specifics can then be examined. The decision about which patient is to receive treatment is necessarily difficult. Different systems of evaluation have been developed. However, a demonstrated shortfall in a capability that threatens the lives and welfare of patients, will aid the process of macro-allocation. There is an obvious relationship between the two. In the meantime, criteria have to be selected and applied. That means choices.

The selection of patients has an immediate and vivid moral aspect. Some of the early examples showed a bias towards certain types of patients, generally those with stable and socially productive backgrounds. Clearly the selection then was done on largely utilitarian grounds. Examples of this are seen in the initial kidney dialysis treatments. The importance of the social value and hence the return to society possible from each candidate was noted. It helped if a patient was married with a family, young and in gainful and significant employment. This may well be a valid allocation of scarce resources, but it involves judgements of value based entirely on utilitarian criteria. This methodology of decision making may be challenged as a thoroughly unethical procedure.

Other factors that may be considered include the one of medical need. The individual whose need is greatest should receive the treatment. This is a principle that appeals to the tradition of natural justice. However, it may not be the most efficient use of resources. Future prospects and prognosis may be particularly bleak in an individual whose need is greatest. By treating him, someone else whose future was brighter may be irreparably compromised.

Morality is not a tidy nor easy business. Consider the common temptation to use age as one of the criteria in any selection process. The intention is to concentrate on the younger candidates. Supporting this is the contention that their life expectancy is much greater and, therefore, there would be a better return on the investment. This argument ignores the natural justice of demonstrated medical need and may well select someone who does not fulfil utilitarian criteria either. In effect it makes a virtue out of youth.

It then becomes advantageous to be young if such treatment is necessary. The element of fortune is introduced. Many selection methods have adopted this principle in its entirety. A lottery is organised and a random allocation is made. This clearly obviates the difficulty of the other methods. It seems to have a degree of acceptability about it as well. Certainly one of its effects is to even out the social background of chosen patients. The intention is to avoid hard moral choices by electing to settle them by the intervention of chance. There may be some point in this exercise when choosing between two equally deserving cases. It eases the job of doctors caught in these invidious positions, and some might contend that it resolves an irreconcilable problem. However, a more general usage of chance as a system of selection poses significant ethical questions. Random allocation does not meet any or even recognise moral criteria in patient selection. The roll of the dice decides.

This cuts to the heart of the matter. Should moral concerns affect the provisions of health care? I have argued that, because of the nature of patient–doctor consultations, there has to be a moral aspect. This imposes additional burdens on the practitioner but is an unavoidable part of the vocation. Many predicaments arise but a firm moral base and integrity are essentially components of caring. The practice of medicine is made both difficult and rewarding by the involvement with other people's lives. At the macro-allocation level the dynamics of social action push criteria towards utilitarianism. This results in the individual doctor doing the best for his patient within constraints set by society. This is the accumulative end point of professional ethical codes, government legislation and the popular conscience. It is surely right that this should be so, and it is supremely moral that it is.

Notes

1. B. G. Myerhoff and W. R. Larson, 'The Doctor as Culture Hero: The Routinization of Charisma', *Human Organization* (1965) vol. 24, pp. 188–91.
2. A. Lewis, 'Health as a Social Concept', *British Journal of Sociology* (1953) vol. 4, pp. 109–24.
3. T. McKeown, *The Origins of Human Disease* (Oxford: Basil Blackwell, 1988) pp. 191–2.
4. B. Russell, *A History of Western Philosophy* (London: Unwin, 1988) pp. 744–7.
5. E. Butler, and M. Pirie, *The Health Alternatives* (London: Adam Smith Institute, 1988) pp. 1–9.

3 Values in Diagnosis

Richard Bentall

Ethical issues in medicine have become an increasingly common topic of philosophical inquiry for a number of reasons.[1] First, moral philosophers have felt the need to demonstrate the relevance of their work to real life problems. Secondly, there has been a growing awareness, both within the medical and related professions and without, that moral judgement plays an important role in clinical practice. Thus, physicians and surgeons may face such dilemmas as whether or not to give oral contraceptives to young girls, or whether or not to turn off the life support machine that is maintaining the vital functions of a brain dead individual. Thirdly, it may be argued that intelligent laypeople are increasingly inclined to question the autocratic 'wisdom' that has sometimes been the hallmark of the clinician's interactions with his or her clients, and are demanding a say in what doctors do to them 'for their own good'.

In response to these observations, some clinicians have expressed reservations about the emergent discipline of philosophical medical ethics.[2] The arguments that have sometimes been made in this respect have been summarised as follows: while ethical issues may be of importance in some areas of medicine, the ideal education in medical ethics is obtained by learning to be a good doctor and by the development of good character, virtue and integrity.[3] A second, not unrelated claim is that, while moral decisions may play a role in clinical practice, philosophical medical ethics is all too subjective a discipline to provide clear guidelines for medical practitioners.[4] The effect of these arguments is to downgrade the role of moral judgement in medicine and to suggest that, where moral judgements are required, they are best left to competent medical practitioners.

In this essay, an attempt will be made to evaluate the importance of moral judgement in clinical practice, bearing these claims in mind. It will be argued that moral concerns will always be implicated in health care as a matter of logical necessity, and that, for various reasons, these concerns cannot be exclusively the province of medical practitioners. Moreover, it will be argued that the failure to recognise the role of moral concerns in health care has resulted in certain important moral judgements masquerading as 'facts'. Finally, it will be shown that the roles played by the caring professions in society at large are open to moral evaluation, requiring that philosophical medical ethics cannot be a discipline internal to medicine.

The examples used when discussing these issues will for the most part be taken from the domain of psychiatric health care, reflecting the author's own experience and education. However, the issues themselves are applicable to all areas of health care.

MORAL JUDGEMENT AND THE 'FACTS'

Moral judgement is involved when a decision has to be made and there is a conflict of interest, so that the question of what ought to be done is raised. Decisions of this sort are encountered very frequently in all types of clinical practice so that even a partial list of examples requires a book length treatment.[5] Broadly speaking, these decisions seem to occur on two levels of scale – decisions about particular aspects of clinical practice (e.g. 'Compared to the alternatives is a prefrontal leucotomy the best treatment for this patient?') and decisions about what ought to be done on a more macrosocial level (e.g. 'What proportion of the health-care budget should be set aside for the prevention, rather than treatment, of disease?'). At both levels, attempts may be made to resolve the problems these kinds of questions raise by relating the conditions under which a decision is required to more general moral principles. Principles that have been evoked for this purpose include the deontological requirement that health-care professionals, politicians and administrators should have regard for other persons, and consequentialist or utilitarian arguments to the effect that moral decisions should be judged by their consequences. Often, these two types of principles lead to the same broad conclusions, although this is not always the case.[6]

A crucial point that must be recognised at once is that the very nature of the provision of health care means that these kinds of decisions cannot be avoided. Whereas it is possible to imagine a health-care system with values different from our own, it is no more possible to imagine a health-care system with no moral values than it is to imagine a married bachelor. Even a health-care system run entirely on the lines of *laissez-faire* capitalism (which is approximated by the health-care system of some countries), and in which people buy or are unable to buy medical attention at prices determined by market forces, has values – the values associated with the profit motive, social Darwinism and so on. And if asked to justify such a system, the health-care practitioners involved might talk about 'the greater good' served by economic incentives, that State interference in private affairs is morally wrong, or that people who are 'too lazy' to support themselves do not deserve the benefits of health care. (These views are not held by the author.)

Even if we can conceive of a health-care system in which there is no limit to the resources that can be drawn upon (perhaps approximated by the health-care system of a society far in the future) moral problems would still be encountered and moral decisions would still be required. For example, given the availability of every possible treatment for a particular condition, it would still be necessary to decide which treatment is best. Moral decisions will therefore always play a role in medical practice; this is a logical requirement that follows whenever there is more than one alternative course of action that can be pursued.

It can be shown that this requirement runs deeper than mere definition by examining the arguments about the appropriate education in medical ethics alluded to above. The claim that a good medical education is sufficient in this respect would seem to boil down to two parts: the view that the moral component in any medical decision is relatively straightforward, and the view that the factual component is so complex that it precludes the involvement of the medically uninitiated in the decision making process.

Of course, it is often all too easy to make a moral decision; many people do so without a moment's reflection, indeed without realising that this is what they are doing. It is possible that the unreflective way in which some people make such judgements has contributed to the appeal of moral philosophies which equate moral decisions with preference[7] or biological necessity.[8] On a more lengthy examination, however, it appears that our unreflective moral judgements are often unreliable. Such judgements have often justified a variety of unsavoury practices which, on subsequent analysis, have proved morally reprehensible. (An example in this respect would be the persecution of minority groups, such as blacks in the southern states of the USA, and Jews in Germany, on the grounds of supposed inferiority). Once the unreliability of these judgements is revealed, it is clear that they must be evaluated against the kind of more general moral principles referred to above. Unfortunately, the moral principles themselves sometimes lead to counterintuitive decisions (for example, when utilitarian considerations lead to the abandonment of principles of justice).[9] Moreover, sometimes moral principles are in conflict. We may object to the compulsory detention of psychiatric patients on the grounds of respecting persons; on the other hand we may feel that detaining such patients is for the greater good. Such moral dilemmas reveal the complexity of moral problems. Sometimes the analysis of such dilemmas, by revealing the issues involved, will lead to agreement about the correct course of action to take. Sometimes, it will not (thus lending apparent support to those who argue that philosophical medical ethics is 'all too subjective' to be of any use). Even when analysis does not lead to resolution, however, it usually reveals issues of which the participants in the dilemma were not aware. By doing so, it maps out the precise 'logical geography' of the dilemma, and of the disagreement between the various protagonists.

As well as mapping out disagreement, the appeal to general moral principles has a second consequence. These principles do not apply exclusively to medicine – they are guidelines for evaluating conduct in all walks of life. Because they apply equally to the domains of law and multinational business, to the conduct of soldiers, housepersons and even philosophers, they cannot be considered purely from the perspective of medicine. Everyone, whether doctor, patient or not, has a 'stake' in these principles and everyone, at least potentially, has something to say about their application. Whereas a doctor might be optimally placed to provide an opinion about the effects of chlorpromazine on brain dopamine levels (although even this is dubious, for pharmacologists could probably claim greater expertise), given a known outcome of chlorpromazine medication, the question of whether this outcome is morally good is open to debate at all levels of society.

This returns us to the argument downgrading the role of philosophical medical ethics alluded to above. The second part of this argument suggests that the factual component of any medical decision is either entirely sufficient to make the decision, or so complex as to be beyond the competence of the medically unqualified. Of course, the question of whether moral decisions can be derived from statements of fact has been extensively debated among moral philosophers. A commonly held view is that they cannot. Thus

Hare[10] claims that the discovery that conclusions containing 'ought' cannot be derived from premises containing 'is' is one of the most important made by moral philosophers. More recently, this view has been challenged, notably by Philippa Foot.[11] From the point of view of the present discussion, a significant aspect of this debate is that it cannot be resolved by reference to 'is' statements, but must be debated by reference to the logic surrounding the language of morals; a physician wishing to avoid philosophical analysis by claiming that he could derive his clinical decisions from the 'facts' about his patients would have to enter the discourse of philosophical analysis to justify doing so. (This ignores the difficult question of how he would gain objective and unprejudiced access to the 'facts' in any case.)

In reality, no-one doubts that the 'facts' are relevant to moral decisions and certainly empirical issues are of central significance to by far the majority of decisions made by medical practitioners. The question then arises: is the undoubted complexity of these issues sufficient to limit ethical decision making to qualified medical practitioners? In answer to this, it should be noted that 'facts' are not the unique possession of any particular group within society. One function of a medical qualification is to provide a guarantee of a minimum level of medical competence in the holder. This does not imply that those without a medical qualification are necessarily incompetent to understand medical information. (In some cases, to be discussed in more detail at the end of the essay, other professions, particularly the scientific disciplines allied to medicine, may have more competence. For example, it is not unknown to see a 'doctor' appearing on television to discuss some aspect of, say, social psychology in an uninformed manner). Even persons lacking any education in science or medicine may be capable of understanding the issues, once explained. And given that such people have a right to be involved in moral-medical decision making for the reasons outlined above, there is a clear moral requirement for medical practitioners and other clinicians to be accountable and explain their actions. The most obvious example of this requirement concerns the goals of treatment. For example, Mark and Ervin[12] have suggested the treatment of aggressive behaviour by surgery to anatomically and physiologically normal brains, a proposal that has implications for all members of society. Similarly, the known outcome of treatments is an aspect of medicine that laypersons might expect to be informed about. For example, it has recently been revealed that several types of psychotropic medication have very serious undesirable side effects, suggesting that these drugs may have been overprescribed relative to their benefits and that non-medical remedies for psychological distress might be more appropriate.[13] Whereas it may be unreasonable to expect laypersons to understand the precise scientific rationale for a particular treatment technique, it is not unreasonable that they be given information about the goals of treatment and the expected results in order to evaluate its desirability, both with respect to an individual case and also with respect to the treatment's macrosocial implications.

To summarise the argument so far, it seems clear that moral issues are crucially and unavoidably important in health care, and that competence to weigh these issues is not restricted to the medically qualified. Unfortunately, these issues have not always received the attention that they have deserved and we shall now turn to what happens when they are not considered.

TWO PROBLEM CASES OF MENTAL DISORDER

In the above discussion, the relationship between moral judgements and 'facts' was briefly considered. It seems clear that, whether or not moral conclusions can be derived from factual premises, an important distinction must be drawn between statements of fact and statements of moral evaluation. Even if the latter can be shown to flow from the former, they are not identical. A moral evaluation contains an explicit recipe for action whereas a statement of fact, on its own, does not. Given that moral judgements play an important role in health care, but that explicit moral debate occupies a relatively small part of the public and professional time devoted to health care, it might be asked how the moral issues are dealt with in practice. In some cases, of course, overworked clinicians are left wrestling with their consciences as they attempt to come to grips with problems that they know are primarily ethical rather than scientific. In other cases, however, a kind of logical sleight of hand occurs, in which moral judgements, implicitly accepted by nearly all concerned, masquerade as 'facts'. Such a false assignment of judgements belonging to the domain of morals to the domain of 'facts' constitutes an example of what Gilbert Ryle has termed a 'category' mistake, akin to looking for a team spirit on a cricket pitch in the belief that it somehow belongs to the logical category of physical objects such as bats, stumps and the cricket ball.[14]

Some of the most striking examples of such errors can be found in psychiatric health care. Psychiatry is in fact a particularly suitable object of moral scrutiny for a number of reasons. The theoretical foundations and practice of psychiatric medicine have come under considerable attack in the past two or three decades. These attacks have been from various sources – from psychiatrists who believe that psychiatry is a pseudoscience which has very little to do with medicine[15] and is inherently dehumanising;[16] from the rival profession of clinical psychology which has emerged since the end of the Second World War,[17] which, according to at least one eminent psychiatrist is attempting to take over the assets of 'Psychiatry Limited'[18] and which advocates the use of radically different (i.e. non-medical) concepts in order to understand madness;[19] from sociologists who view the mentally ill as social deviants and who claim that psychiatrists are agents of the state;[20] from social historians who have analysed the way in which the medical profession made an unwarranted claim of expertise about madness in the eighteenth and nineteenth centuries;[21] and finally from lawyers, politicians and civil rights activists and, indeed, psychiatrists themselves, who have become concerned about the way in which psychiatry has been used to justify the curtailment of the civil liberties of selected individuals both in the West[22] and in other parts of the world.[23] Because of the persistence of these (converging) assaults, it is perhaps fair to say that psychiatry has suffered more at the hands of its critics than any other branch of medicine. Indeed, whereas there are psychiatrists who have thought fit to label themselves as 'anti-psychiatrists', there are no 'anti-gynaecologists', 'anti-pharmacologists', or 'anti-cardiac surgeons'. In general medicine, although particular issues about the provision of health care (e.g. overprescription, early resort to the knife, dehumanising methods of childbirth) have been subject to hot dispute, in psychiatry it is the whole conceptual framework of the discipline that has been challenged.

One repeatedly addressed issue concerns the moral and scientific status of psychiatric 'caseness'. What exactly makes someone a psychiatric case? Can caseness be determined purely on objective grounds or are moral criteria relevant? In order to answer this question, it will be helpful to consider two cases encountered by the author in his work as a clinical psychologist. These cases are by no means remarkable: one was encountered in outpatient practice, the other in a forensic setting. Names and identifying features of each case have been disguised.

Gillian was a 38-year-old woman referred by a general practitioner following a thirteen-year history of depression and anxiety. She had twice been seen by consultant psychiatrists and, following a poor response to tricyclic medication, refused to receive further psychiatric attention. (It is surprisingly common for clinical psychologists to be referred individuals who have first failed to respond to psychiatric intervention.) The author accepted Gillian for treatment with the intention of using cognitive therapy,[24] a form of psychotherapy which has repeatedly been shown to be superior to medication in the treatment of unipolar depression.[25] Briefly, the theoretical rationale of cognitive therapy is that disturbed affect results from holding 'irrational' hypotheses about the world (usually the belief that the world is a bad or evil place, and that the patient is doomed to a life of moral and material inadequacy). The task of the cognitive therapist is to engage the patient in a 'Socratic dialogue', attempted in a spirit of 'collaborative empiricism', so that the hypotheses underlying the disturbance can be tested and, hopefully found false.

Progress in cognitive therapy normally takes a matter of a few months. After a year of almost weekly sessions, however, the author was making no headway. It appeared to the therapist that Gillian, an intelligent under-achiever, was better at the 'Socratic dialogue' than the therapist. After sessions, the exhausted therapist would find himself remarking to his colleagues that 'reverse cognitive therapy' seemed to be occurring. As the patient increasingly convinced the therapist of the accuracy of her world view, the therapist became more and more depressed.

Matters came to a crisis when the patient found the therapist's telephone number and rang up one night, threatening suicide. Faced with the prospect of having a psychiatrist commit the patient to hospital and thus admitting failure, the therapist turned to a wiser colleague who, schooled in family therapy and systems theory, suggested that a 'paradoxical' intervention[26] might be appropriate. Depression might have a function for Gillian. Whereas poor self-esteem seemed to be central to her condition, she appeared to be defending herself from a further loss of self-esteem by 'defeating the therapist at his own game', just as she had defeated all previous help. If encouragement to see the bright side of life was having no effect, perhaps encouragement to see the grim side of life might.

Later that night, the therapist made a domiciliary visit to Gillian and nervously suggested to her that he had completely misunderstood her condition, and that she had a *need* to be depressed in order to keep people interested in her. It was not surprising therefore that his attempts to relieve her depression were making her worse. Unfortunately, the therapist had become so depressed by his failure to help her that he would be unable to see her for at least two weeks (the minimum time recommended to allow a paradoxical message to take effect).

Two weeks later, Gillian dramatically announced that she was 'cured'. The therapist duly disclaimed any responsibility, restated his incompetence, and predicted that the improvement would not last. Over the next few months, as the therapist made further bleak predictions, Gillian began to go out in the evenings, started an evening class to improve her qualifications, and began dating for the first time since her divorce. Her mood, initially euphoric, settled at a normal level and eventually she 'discarded' her therapist, saying that she no longer needed his help.

The second case is as follows: Peter was a not very bright 32-year-old man, with a history of child molesting. Although he was a persistent offender, he had never threatened harm to any of the young boys he assaulted (his modus operandi was to bribe them with sweets). He had frequently been in hospital. After his last discharge he had obtained a labouring job which he had successfully maintained until he was caught having sexual intercourse with an (apparently consenting) 12-year-old boy. On conviction he was given a three-year sentence.

He received no parole. A few days before his sentence would have been over he was interviewed by a prison psychiatrist who judged him to be suffering from a psychopathic disorder. He was transferred to a Special (i.e. secure) Hospital, where he remains today, two years later. In the hospital he has received no treatment of any significance. The psychiatric staff have no medication they can offer him to alter his sexual preferences, and he shows no other signs of mental disorder. The psychology staff feel that the conditions of the institution make psychological intervention well nigh impossible, although the available research indicates that sexual reorientation programmes carried out in the community can sometimes be successful.[27]

Many of the issues raised by Gillian's case are explicitly in the domain of morals. Gillian had a different world view to the author, therefore she was depressed. But was that world view wrong? The cognitive theory of depression, which is the rationale for cognitive therapy, seems to assume that Gillian's views about the world were somehow irrational. This is what led her to be a psychiatric case. However, as the psychologist Michael Mahoney has observed, there seems to be nothing more inherently 'rational' about having an optimistic view of life, 'It's just more pleasant, that's all'.[28]

Some of the issues raised by the case of Peter are rather different. On whose behalf was the psychiatrist, who interviewed Peter in prison, making his diagnosis? Given that the prospects of successful 'treatment' for Peter were grim (and that he did not want treating anyway) was his transfer to a Special Hospital more akin to punishment (without limit of time) than therapy? As in the case of Gillian, however, the question of 'caseness' appears to be particularly important. What made Peter a psychiatric case? Was his diagnosis a scientific judgement or a moral verdict?

THE CASE AGAINST CASENESS

A person usually becomes a psychiatric case by receiving a psychiatric diagnosis. Diagnosis, in turn, is usually regarded as a relatively objective procedure, so that diagnostic uncertainty is typically blamed on a lack of scientific information that can be remedied by empirical research.[29] However, as Reich[30] points out, diagnosis should be the focus of any consideration of the ethics of psychiatry because this one act sustains all the powers, institutions and technologies of psychiatric medicine. Psychiatric diagnosis is therefore ethically problematic because of its consequences for the patients, which on occasion (for example, in the case of Peter) can be extreme. But psychiatric diagnosis has been thought ethically problematic for a second reason that is not considered by Reich, namely because, so critics such as Thomas Szasz would argue,[31] the diagnostic label amounts to a moral judgement (of a pejorative nature) rather than a scientific judgement. The distinction between these two issues is important because, without it, the question of the ethics of diagnosis reduces to the question of how to avoid its misapplications and its undesirable consequences. Thus Reich argues that, 'If enough is really known about mental disorders to be able to categorise them, and if such categorisation does indeed represent a scientifically based or at least pragmatically useful professional activity, then the ethical concerns must be the actual or potential misapplication of diagnostic categories to persons who do not deserve them.' Although the term deserve was probably not meant to be significant here, its presence is telling. What kind of people, precisely,' deserve' psychiatric diagnoses?

This problem has been in existence since medical men first made their claim of expert knowledge about madness. For example, Eysenck quotes the case of Dr Samuel Cartwright,[32] an early American physician, who characterised a disease, *drapatomania*, as a product of weak-mindedness in negro slaves. Its main symptom was 'running away from captivity'. Great Britain has not been free from this kind of obvious misapplication of medical concepts: in the early 1970s scores of old ladies who had originally been certified for having illegitimate children, were found on the back wards of British mental hospitals.[33] However, the most famous recent example of this sort has been the use of the diagnosis 'sluggish schizophrenia' to justify the detention of Soviet dissidents in mental hospitals.[34]

The way in which diagnostic categories can shift with a change in the ethical climate is illustrated by the response of American psychiatrists to changes in the public perception of homosexuality. In the 1970s, during the development of the third edition of the American Psychiatric Association's *Diagnostic and Statistical Manual* (DSM-III), gay rights activists campaigned for homosexuality to be no longer listed as a form of mental disorder. In a national APA meeting, psychiatrists were asked to vote on the issue and homosexuality – which had appeared in (DSM-II) – was voted out of the manual. However, a compromise amendment, proposed by Dr Robert Spitzer (an influential diagnostician) was adopted with the consequence that 'sexual orientation disturbance' (characterised as unhappiness with one's sexual orientation) appeared in its place.[35] The dramatic image of physicians voting a disease out of existence should not lead us to believe that homosexuality represents a unique example. Should there be a significant change in the political climate of the Soviet Union, we might expect 'reformism' no longer to appear as a symptom in the Moscow School of Psychiatry's criteria for 'sluggish schizophrenia'.

An important consideration concerns the meanings of the terms 'disease' and 'illness'. Szasz has argued that mental illness is not really illness because no underlying pathology has been identified. According to Szasz, the label 'illness' amounts to a category mistake that has the functions of obscuring a moral judgement and maintaining psychiatrists as covert social control agents. Wing,[36] on the other hand, has argued that many physical illnesses do not have known biological substrates and that, a better criterion of disease is the existence of a cluster of traits that tend to occur together and for which there is evidence to suggest biological causation. Wing argues that these criteria are satisfied with respect to 'schizophrenia' although a number of other commentators, including Sarbin and Manusco[37] and the author[38] have claimed, on the basis of careful reviews of the evidence, that this is not in fact the case.

A slightly different approach to this problem has recently been proposed by Radden.[39] Radden has argued that the disease model of madness is inappropriate precisely because it is insufficient to justify our ethical intuition that mentally disordered individuals are not responsible for their (sometimes criminal) actions. On the basis of Foucault's social history of psychiatric ideas,[40] Radden claims that before the disease model became widely accepted there was a brief period in which madness was regarded as a loss of reason. Radden claims that this idea has more desirable ethical implications for mad people and that it should be revived. Unfortunately, Radden's analysis leaves in question a crucial issue: whether our intuitions about the moral culpability of mad people are valid. Such intuitions have been used by psychiatrists in order to justify the way in which mentally disordered individuals are routinely deprived of their liberties (for example, with respect to determining their own treatment). Are all mad people so lacking in reason that they really have no idea what is in their own interest? (And, in any case, if this was so, would this justify professional people deciding such issues for them?).

A crucial source of misunderstanding in this debate is posed starkly by the title of Sarbin and Manusco's book *Schizophrenia: Diagnosis or Moral Verdict?* As Sidgwick has pointed out,[41] all diagnoses are made against a background of moral considerations. Appendicitis is an illness, not only because it consists of a cluster of traits of biological origin but also because it is *bad* for people. Viewed from the vantage point of an alien intelligence AIDS is merely the manifestation of a micro-organism (HTLV-III) which has successfully found an evolutionary niche. From this viewpoint, a more correct question to ask is whether, in *addition* to being a moral verdict, schizophrenia – or any other psychiatric diagnosis – amounts to a valid scientific entity. On this account, it has been possible to abuse the concept of mental illness, not because it is morally loaded (all diagnoses are morally loaded), but because clinicians have incorrectly believed that, in addition to being moral verdicts, their diagnoses correspond to scientific facts.

This much is implicit in Reich's account of the way in which psychiatric diagnosis has been abused in the Soviet Union. The concept of 'sluggish schizophrenia' was originated not in order to persecute dissidents, but because the Moscow school of psychiatrists felt that a broad definition of schizophrenia was necessary to take into account mild or borderline conditions. Such borderline conditions have in fact been included in DSM-III under the title of 'schizotypal personality disorder'. The proposal that definitions of schizophrenia should take into account such borderline states resulted, in turn, from the failure of research to establish a valid schizophrenia syndrome.[42]

Not surprisingly, given the poor validity of many psychiatric diagnoses, the borderline between madness and sanity is often difficult to determine. This has been particularly the case in respect to individuals such as Peter who persistently offend against society's rules. Whereas they present no obvious signs of psychopathology (disturbance of affect, thinking or perception) their failure to learn from experience leads to the intuitive assumption that there must be 'something wrong' with them. Thus the psychopath is regarded as presenting a 'mask of sanity'[43] and extensive efforts have been made to identify personality correlates of this form of 'disorder'.[44]

On a more everyday level, however, the distinction between sanity and madness can be difficult to determine. To be classified as a psychiatric case, a person has to pass through a series of 'filters'.[45] The person, or members of the immediate family, have to recognise unusual behaviour which they must attribute to psychological disorder, they must take their 'problem' to a general practitioner who must agree with their verdict and refer the patient to a psychiatrist or a psychologist. Even at this stage, the psychiatrist or psychologist may decide that the patient is not mentally disturbed and may recommend alternative approaches to relieving the distress of the patient and his or her family (e.g. taking a holiday). Whereas symptomatic variables may partially determine progression through this filtering system it is apparent that these are not the only factors involved. Research has consistently shown that psychopathology, as defined as symptoms potentially treatable by psychiatric or psychological methods, are extremely common in the community – present in as many as 50 per cent of the population in the case of mild anxiety or depression.[46] Even comparatively severe psychiatric symptoms are reported by a substantial minority of 'normal' individuals.[47] The cut-off point between madness and normality would thus seem arbitrary, and the prospect of a psychiatric service designed to catch and treat all 'mental illness' would seem to be an impossibility.

If moral evaluation is implicitly involved in determining psychiatric caseness, it might be asked whether the same is true for the diseases and illnesses of general medical practice. It is clear that Sidgwick's observations about the logic of diagnosis apply equally to conditions of known physical causation. moreover, in the case of systemic diseases such as essential hypertension no clear dividing line between normal and abnormal functioning can be determined. (Cases of hypertension consist of the tail of a normal distribution of blood pressures.) Anthropological data indicates important cultural differences in the way that people interpret their symptoms[48] and sociological research also indicates that a variety of demographic and social variables determine which individuals out of the enormous majority who are unwell present for medical help.[49] Still, it might be asked, can examples of morally contentious criteria for caseness, similar to those encountered in psychiatry, be identified in general medicine?

The most obvious contenders for this role concern individuals who are apparently well but who nonetheless are regarded as 'patients'. Pregnant women are a case in point. Pregnancy is a normal biological process, yet the progressive 'medicalisation' of this process has created conditions for the pregnant woman that are not very dissimilar to those that apply to the psychiatric patient. Statutes in most western countries dictate that a woman may not give birth without the attendance of a qualified doctor or midwife. Often, the pregnant woman has little or no control over the way in which she gives birth, the options available to her being determined by the standards of practice advocated by a small group of professional people (usually men). When these standards are challenged, the reaction of the medical professionals has been to oppose any changes in current practice. The unedifying disputes surrounding the recent suspension of an obstetrician in London reflect these disagreements.

A second example of 'caseness' which is morally questionable concerns unfortunate individuals who are serum-positive for HTLV-III, the virus that causes acquired immune deficiency syndrome. As the blood test for HTLV-III only detects anti-bodies to the virus, it only indicates whether the person concerned has come into contact with it, not whether the virus remains in his or her blood. The social consequences of being found HTLV-III anti-body positive are severe (e.g. loss of job, inability to get a mortgage) and yet the available evidence indicates that, outside certain high-risk groups (homosexuals who practice anal sex and drug addicts who share needles), AIDS is a highly *uninfectious* disease. Nonetheless, the detection of HTLV-III anti-body positive individuals is considered a priority by health-care professionals.

Finally, of course, there is the example of those healthy people who persist in consuming excessive quantities of non-prescribed drugs such as alcohol or heroin. Although these types of individuals have often been regarded as in need of health care, and have sometimes been coerced into receiving 'treatment', many observers have claimed that attempts to solve their problems should be social or even penal in nature.[50]

CONCLUSIONS

Ethical dilemmas are so common in medicine that it can plausibly be argued that every medical decision has an ethical component. The decision to give an infected child penicillin involves not only the scientific judgement that penicillin will, in all probability, reduce the infection with minimal side-effects, but also the ethical judgement that this is a desirable goal which can be achieved in no better way. It has been argued that moral issues cannot be avoided in medicine, that they are of importance to everyone and are not the province of medical practitioners alone, and that when ignored they lurk in the body politic of health care disguised as other (usually empirical) issues. To demonstrate this latter point, criteria for psychiatric caseness were considered as an example.

One of the issues to emerge from the above discussion concerns the enormous power that the health-care professions wield within society. Often this power is implicit and manifests itself in the way that medicine and allied disciplines use their 'clout' to influence public opinion. An enormous prestige surrounds medicine, supported by the public perception that medical practitioners have control over death. (This perception may not be entirely accurate.[51] Health-care professionals, particularly doctors, have a privileged position in our society. It thus follows that they have an interest in maintaining this position. In closing, it will be worthwhile considering this issue, which presents a final and most persuasive reason for believing that medical ethics cannot be left to the doctors.

Medical professionals are not the only people who know about helping people with problems. It is true that they have certain skills that they acquire in their training but it is also true that they lack certain skills because of their training. It is again in the field of psychiatry that this observation is most telling. As a number of authors have pointed out, the psychiatrist has an embarrassing lack of unique skills in either the understanding or treatment of madness.[52] Yet the prevailing view that madness is a medical phenomenon maintains medical practitioners in their dominant role in psychiatric services. A case can be made for the argument that this is detrimental to patients as it has led to an excessive reliance on medical (mainly pharmacological) methods of treatment, rather than on psychosocial alternatives that are as cost effective, if not more cost effective, and which have fewer iatrogenic implications. In response to challenges of prevailing practices from other professions, notably clinical psychology, the response from psychiatrists has been to try and limit the influence of the other professions. Until the Trethowan Report of 1977, general practitioners were prevented from referring patients directly to psychologists, and psychiatrists, and psychiatrists still discourage them from doing so in some areas.[53] In the United States similar attempts to prevent psychologists from working directly with patients led to the American Psychological Association taking successful legal action against the American Psychiatric Association under federal trade legislation.[54]

Klass has cited similar examples from other areas of health-care practice, notably pharmocology.[55] (Klass argues that the skills of most pharmacists, working as dispensing chemists, are considerably underutilised and this is a historical result of the way in which medical practitioners have sought to limit the pharmacist's role.)

It is above all because the medical profession (and all other health-care professions, including clinical psychology and pharmacy), are social forces which have interests to defend that their roles within society are open to ethical examination. In as much as medical ethics is absorbed within the practice of medicine and used to justify existing practices it will be a force of reaction and, paradoxically, will lead to worse rather than better health care. Philosophical medical ethics must distance itself a step from medicine, indeed from health care as a whole, before considering its subject matter. Philosophical medical ethics is 'medical' only because of the direction in which it looks, not because of the direction from which it comes.

Notes

1. J. Dawson and M. Phillips, M. *Doctor's Dilemmas* (Brighton: Harvester, 1985).
2. J. Watt, *British Medical Journal* (1980) vol. 281, pp. 1687–80; J. D. Swales, *Journal Medical Ethics* (1982) vol. 8, pp. 117.
3. R. Gillon, *British Medical Journal* (1985) vol. 290, pp. 1497–8.
4. R. Gillon, ibid., pp. 1574–5.
5. R. Veatch and R. Branson, *Case Studies in Medical Ethics* (Cambridge, Mass.: Harvard University Press, 1977).
6. T. Beauchamp and J. F. Childress, *Principles of Biomedical Ethics* (Oxford: Oxford University Press, 1980).
7. A. Ayer, *Language Truth and Logic* (Harmondsworth: Penguin, 1971).
8. M. Midgley, *Beast and Man* (Brighton: Harvester Press, 1982).
9. J. J. C. Smart and B. Williams, *Utilitarianism for and against* (Cambridge: Cambridge University Press, 1973).
10. R. Hare, *The Language of Morals* (Oxford: Oxford University Press, 1956).
11. P. Foot, *Virtues and Vices* (London: Basil Blackwell, 1978).
12. V. H. Mark and F. R. Ervin, *Violence and the Brain* (New York: Harper and Row, 1970).
13. D. Hill, *The Politics of Schizophrenia* (American Universities Press, 1984).
14. G. Ryle, *The Concept of Mind* (Harmondsworth: Penguin, 1949).
15. R. D. Laing, *The Politics of Experience* (Harmondsworth: Penguin, 1967).
16. D. Cooper, *Psychiatry and Anti-psychiatry* (London: Paladin, 1977).
17. D. McKay, *Clinical Psychology* (London: Methuen, 1977).
18. A. Clare, *Psychological Medicine*, vol. 9, pp. 387–9.
19. A. Bandura, *Principles of Behaviour Modification* (New York: Rinehart and Winston, 1969).
20. T. Scheff, *Being Mentally Ill* (New York: Aldine, 1966).
21. A. Scull, *Museums of Madness* (London: Penguin, 1979).
22. L. Gostin, *'A Human Condition'*, *MIND* (1976).
23. M. Lader, *Psychiatry on Trial* (Harmondsworth: Penguin, 1977).
24. A. T. Beck, *Cognitive Therapy and Emotional Disorders* (New York: New American Library, 1976).

25. J. M. G. Williams, *The Psychological Treatment of Depression* (Beckenham: Croom Helm).
26. J. Haley, *Problem Solving Therapy* (New York: Harper and Row, 1976). Paradoxical messages are those that have the opposite intention to their explicit content and might therefore be treated as lies, making them of some moral interest in their own right; see S. Bok, *Lying* (Hassocks, Sussex: Harvester Press).
27. G. Abel, *et al.*, 'A community based programme for sexual offenders' (unpublished manual).
28. M. Mahoney, *Cognition and Behaviour Modification* (Ballinger, 1974).
29. R. K. Blashfield, *The Classification of Psychopathology* (New York: Plenum, 1984).
30. W. Reich, in S. Bloch and P. Chodoff (eds), *Psychiatric Ethics* (Oxford: Oxford University Press, 1981).
31. T. Szasz, *The Myth of Mental Illness* (New York: Harper and Row, 1971).
32. H. J. Eysenck, *The Future of Psychiatry* (London: Methuen, 1976).
33. T. Szasz, *The Manufacture of Madness* (London: Routledge, 1976).
34. W. Reich, ibid.
35. R. Bayer, *Homosexuality and American Psychiatry* (New York: Basic Books, 1981).
36. J. K. Wing, *Reasoning about Madness* (Oxford: Oxford University Press, 1978).
37. T. Sarbin and J. C. Manusco, *Schizophrenia: Diagnosis or Moral Verdict* (New York: Pergamon, 1980).
38. R. P. Bentall, in H. F. Jackson and D. Pilgrim, *British Journal of Clinical Psychology* (1988) vol. 27, pp. 303–24, and 329–31.
39. J. Radden, *Madness and Reason* (London: Allen and Unwin, 1985).
40. M. Foucault, *Madness and Reason* (New York: Random House, 1966).
41. P. Sidgwick, *Psychopolitics* (London: Pluto Press, 1982).
42. R. P. Bentall *et al.*, ibid.
43. H. Cleckley, *The Mask of Sanity* (New York: Mosby, 1966).
44. R. Hare and D. Schalling (eds), *Psychopathic Behavior: An Approach to Research* (New York: Wiley, 1978).
45. D. Goldberg and P. Huxley, *Mental Illness in the Community* (London: Tavistock, 1980).
46. R. Cochrane, *Social Creation of Mental Illness* (Longman, 1981).
47. R. Cochrane, ibid.
48. G. Scambler, in D. L. Patrick and G. Scambler (eds), *Sociology as Applied to Medicine* (London: Balliere Tindall, 1982).
49. G. Scambler, ibid.
50. R. Cochrane, in D. Blackman and J. Sanger (eds), *Aspects of Psychopharmocology* (London: Methuen 1985).

51. T. McKeown, *The Role of Medicine* (Oxford: Blackwell, 1979).
52. J. Trethowan, *The Role of the Clinical Psychologist* (DHSS, 1977). See also McKay, ibid.
53. For example, see McKay (ibid.) and Bandura (ibid.) and Blashfield (ibid.).
54. H. Dorken and J. T. Webb, *American Psychologist* (1980) vol. 35, pp. 355–63.
55. A. Klass, *Thar's Gold in Them Thar Pills* (Harmondsworth: Penguin, 1976).

4 Moral Dilemmas in Health Care

Michael Saunders

First, I wish to outline what is happening when one makes a moral judgement as opposed to any other kind of judgement. Normative judgements are not necessarily moral; it depends on the point of view taken. If my wife tells me that I ought to go to London by train rather than car, her reason is that it takes less time. The reason is prudential. When she tells me to wear a matching shirt and tie because the ones I am wearing clash, her judgement is aesthetic. On the other hand, when I am told that I ought to go and see my friend Ron because I had promised to help him over a personal problem with his son, there is an obligation to keep a promise and help someone. This involves a moral obligation rather than a non-moral one.

In a non-moral judgement one takes a calm approach, using reason, impartiality, a willingness to universalise, taking the issue as we find it and attempting to determine what a rational choice would be. In non-moral judgements we evaluate things such as cars, pieces of medical equipment, the relative merits of drugs and works of art. We may refer to such judgements as a good painting or an excellent piece of medical equipment, but we do not mean that such things are morally good or bad; they are neutral in this respect. They are not the kinds of things we would regard as morally good or bad.

When one makes moral judgements in relation to choices between particular actions, we regard certain actions as morally right or wrong; we should still be impartial and rational but we feel a duty to do a certain thing; there is a feeling of 'oughtness' about it. This does not explain why we have such views: that is in the area of metaethics. Apart from cultural and social conditioning and religious beliefs, we may take the view that ultimate moral attitudes are absolutes that are available to everyone to adopt, given the appropriate degree of rationality, or we may regard them as relative values which have no absolute status at all. This might imply that the only reason we regard some judgements and obligations as moral, as opposed to non-moral, is a matter of emotion and feeling or approval and disapproval.

However, in practice we do regard choices as morally right or wrong, good or bad. There is a difference between the obligation to buy a new suit and the duty to go and see my hospital in-patients on a regular basis. Moral issues are important ones which affect the welfare of other humans and sometimes animals and the environment.

To the person untutored in philosophy it seems fairly clear that moral dilemmas occur. A moral dilemma is a situation in which an agent ought to do more than one act but is unable to do so because doing one involves not doing the other, or something about the way the world is prevents both being done. For instance, I ought to maintain patient confidentiality but there are occasions (see below) when I have public responsibility and I ought to disclose information revealed in consultation. In another situation I ought to preserve the lives of a foetus and the mother, but I cannot do both, for the nature of the world at present is that a foetus up to a certain stage of gestation cannot be separated from the mother and survive; so that if the mother must exist without the foetus to remain alive, the foetus will die.

However, although ordinary people are involved in states of perplexity about moral issues, philosophers have debated whether moral dilemmas exist at all. The matter is of some relevance since utilitarian philosophy, which has a powerful influence on health-care decision making, excludes the objective reality of moral dilemmas; it is an answer to them as it cuts through the maze of conflicting principles utilising the one principle of happiness which is related to outcome.

Mill stated that 'unequivocal cases of conflicting obligations' do arise,[1] but that utility may be used as a means of resolving incompatible demands. Thus if there is a moral dilemma as to whether to use a sum of money to open our out-patient neurology physiotherapy service, which has been closed, or provide much needed equipment for the neurological service, utilitarianism can, in theory, solve this problem. Mill accepts that utility may be difficult to apply, but in no other system is there an 'umpire' to adjudicate between conflicting demands.

Hare, who takes a utilitarian approach, recognises that there are apparent moral conflicts.[2] He overcomes this by suggesting that we operate at two levels, the 'intuitive' and the 'critical'. The critical level is the one that has to be used in solving the moral conflicts that are apparent at the intuitive level. At the critical level an action is judged right or wrong on a utilitarian basis. In our ordinary living we operate on a few simple prima facie principles, and we can include beneficence, non-maleficence, justice, truth telling, promise keeping and confidentiality. These principles can conflict in an apparent moral dilemma. At this point one has to return to a 'critical level' of thinking and solve the dilemma by using utilitarian criteria. Thus the dilemma is soluble. Hare writes that 'the intuitive level conflicts are indeed unreasonable, but at the critical level there is a requirement that we resolve the conflict'.[3]

I myself do not find this particularly helpful. Take the following example. A patient is referred to me who is diagnosed as having epilepsy. After investigation the situation is explained to him and he is commenced on treatment. He is advised that he should not drive a car and that he should report his medical condition to the Department of Transport in Swansea. It comes to my attention that he is continuing to drive and when confronted with this, he explains that he lives in the country, there is no other means of transport, and that he will lose his job if he gives up his licence. He points out that his attacks are now controlled and that he cannot afford to be without his licence for two years.

I find there is a conflict between my obligation of confidentiality to this patient and a wider public responsibility to protect the general public from someone who may be unsafe on the roads. The patient is breaking the law and one cannot exclude the possibility of him having an epileptic attack at the wheel of his car and killing himself and others. On the other hand, he is going to lose his job and his family may suffer in various ways if he gives up driving.

Various principles appear to conflict here. There is an obligation of confidentiality towards the patient inherent in the doctor–patient relationship; a duty of beneficence to the patient and society at large; the patient has a right to exercise autonomy with respect to what he does, including breaking the law, if he decides it is in his personal interests to do so. From my point of view the two main principles which conflict are confidentiality on the one hand and public responsiblity or beneficence on the other. I have a duty of confidentiality in respect of my role as a doctor, an office normally associated with such a duty; this conflicts with my duty as a citizen. There might be a conflict with respect to non-maleficence towards the patient, in that by not reporting him I could be responsible for his death; yet this would conflict with the autonomous wishes of the patient.

From the point of view of Hare's intuitive moral dilemma it is clear that I have a problem. I do not really know what to do; either way I am worried about what the outcome will be. If I reported the patient I would feel guilty and have regrets. It I did not report him and, let us assume that no one else knows, I would feel equally bad if something happened.

This kind of dilemma is not resolved for me by any obvious route at the intuitive level. I have not ranked the principles in my own mind. In fact I decide not to report him and have done so in a number of similar situations. Others would disagree. I decide that in my role as a doctor the duty of confidentiality is of great importance. I accept that there are moral arguments the other way and my colleague up the road picks up the telephone and speaks to Swansea. The protection societies have stated that they will defend doctors who report people with epilepsy who drive.

Moral dilemmas, even if they are apparent, do not seem to me to be solved by evidence. Factual information is important, but if one is involved in a conflict of deontological principles, one is not going to change the decision merely on the basis of an unknown outcome or extra evidence. For instance, would I act any differently if the man had frequent fits so that he was a very significant risk? Also, he might not take his drugs. In that more extreme position the risk to the general public is much greater. If I am consistent I must still come to the same decision if I believe that confidentiality is important. At that point one does become very perplexed and worried. Hare would point to the value of the critical level in solving such a dilemma.

In the more extreme case a critical analysis using utilitarian criteria would cause one to conclude that in the extreme case the man should be reported. On the other hand, the weight of evidence in the less severe case is more evenly balanced and one might conclude that the public risk was minimal and that the preservation of confidentiality would maximise the happiness of the man and his family with negligible risk to the general public. Thus Hare might argue that there is no real dilemma if one applies the 'critical' level analysis in such difficult cases. The deontologist caught up in a conflict of principles with no certain ranking order has no solution other than preferring one principle over another. He would normally wish to universalise the principle to apply to other similar cases; and he would not solve the dilemma by reference to evidence although factual data is important in any situation.

One personal feature of the dilemma example I gave was that whichever way I decided, I would feel guilt or concern over the option that could not be followed. As the two 'rights' were in conflict there was an emotional response on my part to the 'ought' that I could not fulfil. I did not abandon it. This seems to me an important feature of a moral conflict. Consider this dilemma. Carol, who is 19, has a rare but relatively benign disorder of muscle tone which several other members of the family have. It is treated by a drug, Levodopa, which is not normally given at this age. She is very well. She becomes pregnant by her boyfriend. She comes to see me, wanting an abortion. She gives the following reasons. First, she does not really want the baby; secondly, she is afraid the drug she is taking will damage it. The drug company confirm that it may be toxic, but they have no data in humans as it is rarely used in people of child-bearing age. Thirdly, she feels that pregnancy may affect her disease and her state of mind. There is little evidence, one way or the other, that this would be the case. The drug can cause altered mood, but she is basically depressed because she has fallen pregnant.

There must be a reasonable chance that the foetus would be quite normal. Carol could stop her medication. It would slow her up, but it would not be catastrophic. There are conflicting duties of beneficence towards Carol, non-maleficence to the foetus. If one holds beliefs about the sanctity of foetal life and not killing foetuses, there would be powerful principles against acting on Carol's wishes. There is the question of Carol's autonomy, but this involves other people as well – the doctors and nurses. In many similar circumstances foetuses are aborted with very little firm evidence that they will be born abnormal or that a reasonable life could not be lived. Should one abort every Down's foetus, every boy conceived by a Duchenne dystrophy carrier on the basis of a 50 per cent chance it might have the disease?

I reluctantly decide to follow the principle of beneficence towards Carol. The point I want to make here is that I feel guilt and regret about the 'ought' of non-maleficence to the foetus. Williams argues that when two moral 'oughts' conflict we act but do not necessarily abandon the other.[4] The conflicting elements are not eliminated. They are not resolved. He calls this a moral 'remainder'. Thus the dilemma exists in that one 'ought' is not rejected, and thus it is not true to say that it did not apply. It has been argued that this regret is not moral in that it represents an emotional response to consequences; however, in some situations regret can be related to a context which is morally regrettable and I would suggest that this is the situation in the above example.

The best argument in favour of moral dilemmas seems to be that there is a plurality of moral principles and that they inevitably conflict on occasions. There is no clear way out of this conflict. Lemmon has stated that an ought statement can be based on a person's status or position,[5] e.g. the doctor's position vis-á-vis his patients' calls for confidentially or on general moral principles. These can conflict. In my example of epilepsy there was a conflict between a duty based on my status as a doctor, and a moral rule of beneficence towards the general public, and the autonomy of persons. One could also say that inherent in the doctor–patient relationship is a promise or commitment to confidentiality. In the example of the pregnant girl there is a conflict of moral principles less clearly related to status or promises.

The conflicting principles in a pluralist theory of moral dilemmas may be resolved in a number of ways. Ross suggests that one principle has the greater 'stringency'.[6] Rawls refers to second order priority principles,[7] i.e. that one principle overrules another. That could mean that one of the conflicting principles does not apply in a case, which would imply that there was no dilemma, or that although it is preferable to follow one principle rather than another, the other still applies, so there is still a dilemma. The conflict is not eliminated. The other view is that the conflicting principles cannot be resolved. The values are 'incommensurable' – a term used by Nagel.[8] There is no resolution of the problem, we come to some mode of action, but it is not a resolution. This has a ring of truth about it to me and certainly seems appropriate to many health-care conflicts.

It has been suggested that there are conditions in which a moral dilemma may occur although there is only one moral value. This could occur with the question of promise keeping, or the saving of innocent lives. We have recently been involved in an outbreak of meningococcal meningitis. Several children have been admitted to the ITU. One could envisage a situation where there was only one bed and respirator available and two people were sent into hospital, both in critical condition. It would seem that the principle of beneficence could not be extended to both. Assuming they both arrived at the same time, in the same condition, Hare might argue that this could be resolved by recourse to a 'critical' evaluation of utility. It could also be argued that one has to save one or the other life and the resulting anguish is not moral.

Although this example is a particularly acute one, it does seem that it is relevant to many moral dilemmas in health care – an obvious example being the recent controversy over paediatric cardiac surgery in Birmingham. It would seem that even if one resolves the conflict by saving one life rather than another, the other 'ought' persists as a moral remainder, and that this is a situation where only one principle is at stake.

Even if one could argue that a dilemma can occur over one principle, that principle has to be one that is a potential source of conflict within itself. This is not the case with utilitarianism, where the principle is that the right action is the one that maximises happiness and that, in theory, need never be a matter of conflict. It would appear that if one accepts the existence of moral dilemmas their resolution is a matter of debate. One could regard the outcome as a mere act of intuition with no ranking process; or more realistically that any principles are 'incommensurable' and one might as well toss a coin. However, one could debate whether when there are two conflicting 'oughts', there is a possibility that one action is still the right one on some rational basis. This would have to involve some kind of ranking system. Is the final 'ought', the action that is done, of a different order to the first 'oughts'? Williams has suggested that this acted upon 'ought' is non-moral – a deliberate 'ought' – thus the dilemma is not solved from a moral outlook. Foot considers that both 'oughts' have a moral meaning.[9] The horns of the dilemma, as in the examples I have given, represent the conflicting moral 'oughts'. The second moral 'ought' what is done, represents the best thing morally – this can be called a must-prescription. This is what is morally best and what must be done. The obvious way this could be understood is through an acceptance of moral pluralism where the first 'oughts' are the conflicting principles and the second 'ought' or must is the action guide.

However, it seems far from clear to me how the must-prescription in a moral dilemma can be arrived at. I am far more inclined to think there is no satisfactory solution to many dilemmas; one just does one's best! In coming to a must-prescription, one would either rely on intuition, or in some ranking of principles. It might be possible to produce a priority principle. It does not have to mean that one principle overrides another in all circumstances. One could say, for instance, that in the case of an abortion where there is weighty evidence that the health of the mother will suffer, beneficence to the mother has to take preference. But this would not be the case in all abortion situations. However, even if one can find situations where it seems possible to rank principles in relation to the particular conditions of a case, it seems likely that this could not always be so and that there are cases in which there is no resolution.

Moral realism seems a difficult view to sustain in the presence of apparently insoluble dilemmas. One could take the view of MacIntyre 'that there is an objective moral order, but our perceptions of it are such that we cannot bring moral truths into complete harmony with each other'.[10] However, Williams suggests that moral dilemmas do not support realism in the sense that if we feel morally obliged to do two conflicting things, then it is not a matter of one being right and the other wrong. We feel regret over the one we did not do. In contrast, Foot has stated that inconsistent statements, as in a conflict of 'musts', cannot both be true – they are not both morally best. Thus, as discussed above, there can only be one must statement, but conflicting horns in the dilemma are possible.

In conclusion, moral dilemmas differ from non-moral conflicts because they are about serious matters that affect human welfare, or involve major issues about animals and the environment. Philosophers have argued as to whether moral dilemmas exist at all. Certainly, utilitarianism, including the variety explored by Hare, seems to preclude real dilemmas. They are only apparent. If one accepts moral dilemmas, they consist of a conflict of moral principles – there are two conflicting 'oughts' representing the horns of the dilemma. There are sound moral arguments for either 'ought'. If we accept that moral dilemmas exist, the perplexity may be solved by intuition, some appeal to 'staging' or ranking or we may accept that the conflicting principles are 'incommensurable'. We may follow Foot and consider that from the conflicting 'oughts' there is a solution, a 'must'; or we may follow Williams and see moral dilemmas related to moral sentiments and continue to express regret about a moral remainder when the other horn of the dilemma has not been abandoned. Whatsoever the situation it is in practice impossible to solve dilemmas by appeal to facts alone.

Notes

1. J. A. Mill, *Utilitarianism in the Utilitarians* (Garden City, New York: Doubleday and Company, 1961) chap. 2, para. 25.

2. R. M. Hare, *Moral Thinking* (Oxford: Oxford University Press, 1981) pp. 25–62.
3. Ibid.
4. R. Williams, 'Ethical Consistency in Problems of the Self', *Philosophical Papers* (Cambridge: Cambridge University Press, 1956–1972) pp. 166–86.
5. J. Lemmon, 'Moral Dilemmas', *Philosophical Review* (1962) vol. 71, pp. 139–58.
6. W. D. Ross, *The Right and the Good* (Oxford: Oxford University Press, 1930) pp. 16–34, 41–2.
7. J. Rawls, *A Theory of Justice* (Oxford: Oxford University Press, 1973).
8. T. Nagel, *The Fragmentation of Value in Mortal Questions* (Cambridge: Cambridge University Press, 1979) pp. 138–41.
9. P. Foot, 'Moral Realism and Moral Dilemma', *The Journal of Philosophy* (1983) vol. 80, pp. 379–98.
10. A. Macintyre, *After Virtue; A Study in Moral Theory* (Notre Dame: University of Notre Dame, 1981) p. 134.

5 Moral Disputes in Health Care

Eve MacGregor

My examination of the nature of moral disputes and their resolution will be conducted in three phases. First, an analysis of what is meant by a 'moral dispute'. Second, an evaluation of utilitarianism and its adequacy as an ethical theory, for if the theory is itself incoherent then it is possible that an appeal to its principles, far from being useful, will not only fail to achieve a satisfactory resolution but will also tend to distort the issues at hand. Third, a more general discussion of the ways in which moral disputes may be resolved. If it can be shown that some moral conflicts are so deep-rooted that resolution is not, perhaps, ever attainable then it would appear that it is unrealistic to expect utilitarian criteria or those of any other theory to resolve them. If however the resolution of moral conflict can be attained in at least some cases, then the efficacy of utilitarian criteria can be compared with that of other possible means of resolution.

I shall try to argue that, in spite of its weaknesses, the utilitarian approach is useful to people making moral choices, e.g. in medical ethical committees and a consideration of 'consequences' is a helpful tool, amongst others for reaching a decision. However I shall also try to show that once a dispute has arisen, and the parties in the dispute are 'locked-in' to their opposing positions, then it sometimes seems that there is very little either can do to resolve their disagreement. Here the utilitarian, like his opponent, may be forced to accept the limitations of his arguments.

I take 'moral disputes' to mean disputes that arise when there is a lack of agreement concerning what is, or was, the right course of action in a situation that requires a moral choice to be made. Different moral theories need not always result in conflict at the level of action. It is possible to reach the same conclusion concerning the morally right course of action from arguments based on conflicting theories; i.e. there is no dispute about what should be done, although the justifications for doing it are different in each case. For example, a utilitarian could agree with a deontologist that a particular foetus should not be aborted: the former arguing that 'continuing this pregnancy will result in a greater balance of happiness over unhappiness than if it were terminated', and the latter that 'this foetus is an innocent human being and killing innocent human beings is wrong'.

However, disputes over issues like abortion and euthanasia do commonly occur. We can compare these disputes about the ethics of the practitioner's actions, with other clinical (and also often complex) disputes that may arise in health care. For example, there may often be dispute about the best way of treating a handicapped neonate in order to aid its survival: what diagnostic tests to run, which drugs to use, which type of operation to perform and when, but the dispute about whether we should even attempt to aid its survival or choose to let it die is a moral one.

In both types of argument the disputants can give reasons for their judgements. But while we can assume that clinical disputes are, at least in theory, capable of resolution, it is more difficult to see what reasons can resolve conflicting moral judgements. For example in a clinical dispute about when to close a spinal lesion 'current statistics show that survival rates are higher if the operation is performed on day X' may be offered. We may reject it and argue, for example, that 'this baby is not yet fit enough for anaesthesia', but at least we can agree what counts as a reason in such a dispute. However in a dispute between the conflicting moral judgements 'this baby should be treated' and 'this baby should be allowed to die' it may be that the disputants will not even admit the relevance of each other's reasons.

Clearly not anything will count as a proper reason in such a dispute. We should regard with horror a consultant who claimed the baby should be allowed to die because 'it has red hair' or 'my surgical team doesn't operate on Fridays – they play golf'. However, even if he says the baby should be allowed to die, because 'its expected quality of life is very poor' he can anticipate considerable frustration in attempting to resolve a dispute with the registrar, who may argue that 'this baby should be treated because all human life should be valued whatever its quality is deemed to be'. The registrar simply does not acknowledge that the idea of 'quality of life' is morally relevant.

Underlying the conflicting moral principles in such a dispute are the particular moral theories of the disputants. I shall next consider utilitarian theory, outline what I consider to be some of its main strengths and weaknesses and then in the light of this assessment and the problems concerning resolution I have referred to above, consider whether an appeal to utilitarian criteria can be at all useful in trying to reach agreement in moral disputes.

A classic statement of utilitarian theory can be found in J. S. Mill's claim that 'actions are right in proportion as they tend to promote happiness, wrong as they tend to produce the reverse of happiness. By happiness is intended pleasure, and the absence of pain; by unhappiness pain and the privation of pleasure'.[1] Later utilitarians have found problems with the idea of 'tendency', for surely a particular act either does or does not cause happiness. They have also pointed out that the implication of 'in proportion to' is that there are 'degrees of rightness' of acts. Thus a revised and more acceptable statement might be 'an act is right if, and only if, there is no other act the agent could have done that results in a greater balance of happiness over unhappiness'. Later theories have also valued other ends as well as 'happiness', e.g. virtue and knowledge, but share the fundamental belief that the rightness or wrongness of an action is determined by the goodness or badness of its consequences. Thus the only reason for an act to be right is its 'utility', i.e. its usefulness for producing good consequences or, dependent on the situation, the least bad ones. This is in contrast to theories that hold that actions can be judged to be right or wrong in themselves, independently of their consequences.

Beauchamp and Childress[2] list five criteria for assessing the adequacy of a moral theory: clarity, internal consistency, completeness, simplicity and its ability to account for 'the whole range of moral experience, including our ordinary judgements'. They suggest we should be suspicious of a theory that yields conclusions totally at odds with ordinary moral consciousness. There do seem to be problems in using 'ordinary moral consciousness' as some kind of critical standard – for if we can rely on it why do we need theories of ethics? However, there can be situations where the answer reached by utilitarian calculation seems to be morally the wrong answer. I shall try to illustrate this later.

There is an obvious appeal in a theory that appears to meet the criteria of simplicity and completeness by giving one general criterion of a morally right action. For the utilitarian, unlike the deontologist, there can be no competing moral claims. The right action is the one that is the best thing to do on the whole and if two actions result in the same utility it cannot matter which he does. 'Justice' and 'duty', for example, are valued for their utility alone. Utilitarianism seems 'tidy'; it appears to offer a definite procedure for making moral choices, and the idea that in order to decide the right course of action we have 'only' to calculate the utilities of the possible alternatives and compare them seems attractive and progressive, for we are not relying on religion, intuition or tradition.

For example, in deciding whether to continue ventilating or 'switch off' a severely brain-injured patient the procedure would be to calculate and compare the sum of benefits for each course of action. The consequences that would need to be considered might include: whether the patient is being denied the chance of recovery, however slight, or risks recovering to become a vegetable, the effect on the patient's relatives and friends, the effect on the morale of the hospital staff, the value of having a machine free for another patient.

Once we start to apply the principle of utility to an actual situation it no longer seems a simple procedure – we have to take into account the likely consequences for all the people who will be significantly affected. If we use the Greatest Happiness Principle then on what grounds do we assume that happiness is a desirable consequence? Mill's argument from his observation that people do in fact desire happiness seems inadequate since people also desire such things as freedom, love and self-expression.

If we extend the idea of happiness to include these, it then becomes difficult to see how we can weigh these happinesses and ascribe some kind of mathematical value to them. Mill distinguishes 'higher' and 'lower' pleasures and tries to evaluate the quality as well as the quantity (intensity and duration) of happiness. But since the experience of happiness is individual how can we agree on a 'quality rating', indeed it does not even seem to make sense to say that one pleasure is 'twice as high in quality' as another. If the ventilator is switched off, how do we compare the relatives' possible sense of relief that the 'worst has happened' with the nurse's relief that she no longer has to monitor that patient, and can have a tea-break instead? Calculations of utility seem to require that this is possible.

Against these objections the utilitarian might wish to argue that the problem of justifying happiness as a desirable consequence is no greater than the problems of justifying the ultimate assumptions of any moral doctrine, e.g. the justification of a theory that depends on a belief in the existence of God. He might also argue that the difficulties in calculating utility are practical rather than conceptual and still claim that if the consequences could be fully worked out we should know what is the right action.

Another objection to utilitarianism arises from a consideration of situations where the application of utilitarian criteria seems to result in an outcome that conflicts with our everyday moral experience. Suppose the patient on the ventilator has no dependants and no relatives or friends who might be upset by his death. And in another ward is a young father with compatible tissue type whose life can be saved only by urgent organ transplant. Utilitarian calculation might lead us to conclude that greater happiness is achieved by saving the young father and we should switch off the ventilator. (We could assume the effect on the staff to be the same for either death!) We now seem to have created a dispute where ordinary moral awareness finds no conflict; we do not deliberately kill patients that we think might recover. Such an action may have considerable utility, but we should still want to call it immoral.

What seems to be absent from utilitarian theory is the claim that people have an intrinsic moral worth that prevents their being used merely as a means to an end. By considering an action only in terms of its consequences utilitarianism fails to consider whether the action itself is morally justifiable. The morality of the action becomes a matter of indifference and our basic moral ideas of, for example, autonomy and integrity can be ignored. Further, it ceases to matter who is doing what to whom as long as the effect on the impersonal sum of utilities is known.

Ian Kennedy quotes an interesting example of the application of utilitarian criteria in an American law case in 1969.[3] The court allowed the removal of a kidney from a 27-year-old man, with a mental age of 6 years, for transplant into his 26-year-old brother, on the grounds that the donor 'was greatly dependent on his brother emotionally and psychologically' and that 'his well-being would be jeopardised more severely by the loss of his brother than the removal of his kidney'. A non-utilitarian would probably want to question the morality of performing this sort of surgery on someone unable to give mature and informed consent.

Rule utilitarianism seeks to avoid such pitfalls of act utilitarianism, by arguing that counter-intuitive acts will not in fact maximise welfare and our calculation of utility must take into account the negative effect of contravening conventional moral principles. But once he starts to consider the imagined consequences of general rules and not the consequences of particular actions the utilitarian seems to be moving away from the advantages originally claimed for utilitarianism.

In reply to his critics, the utilitarian can point to situations where having no regard to the consequences results in a 'moral mess' similar to the ones of which he is often accused. Some utilitarians would accuse the proponents of other doctrines of prejudice and dogma. For example, upholding the principle 'lying is wrong' when a dying child seeks the truth about his condition may also appear to be counter-intuitive.

I have tried to show some of the weaknesses and strengths of the utilitarian approach to making moral choices. I am not sure that the difficulties are so great that we should abandon an examination of consequences altogether when making a moral decision. The utilitarian approach does still seem useful in clarifying what issues are involved. The question that seems to be emerging is whether the principle of utility or indeed any moral principle is useful as a rule for action. J. L. Stocks[4] argues that this approach is misguided and the main task of the philosopher is not to produce rules for moral action and seek 'tidy ethical systems', but rather to reflect on the nature of the moral principles themselves.

Finally the question I wish to answer in this essay is not how useful are utilitarian criteria for making moral choices, but how useful are they for resolving disputes? If we consider generally by what means moral disputes may be resolved then, I suggest, three possibilities are apparent. Firstly, one party could show the other that the whole moral theory on which he bases his choice of action is false and must be abandoned. Secondly, one disputant offers reasons that the other finds convincing, e.g. he forces his opponent to realise that adherence to certain of his moral convictions will have an unacceptable result, or he shows that his opponent has made an erroneous factual judgement in his argument. Thirdly, it is possible that although neither party brings forward any further reasons one party simply 'comes to see' his opponent is right.

The first possibility seems to require that ultimate justification of moral theories is attainable. As stated earlier, there are problems in justifying the Happiness Principle, but so are there problems for the ultimate justification of any moral theory, and if it is the case that a search for an objective theory of ethics is misplaced then it seems unlikely the parties to the dispute will make progress in this area of debate. The second possibility does seem to offer some real hope of resolution. Since a moral dispute is often characterised not only by the particular moral beliefs of the disputants but also by disagreement over the relevant facts, this non-moral element may sometimes be decisive in resolving the dispute. For example, in a dispute about whether we should save lives by providing universal screening for breast cancer or choose to allocate resources to geriatric care, if it could be shown that screening was not in fact effective in detecting malignancies, or was even actually harmful, then the dispute might be resolved. It is interesting that in their campaign for a tightening of the abortion laws Pro-Life now intend to use arguments about the alleged pain felt by the foetus because their arguments based on the sanctity of human life have been ineffective in winning over the Left. However, I suggest this may turn out to be a quasi-factual argument – akin to arguments about the human status of the foetus – since the parties to the dispute may not be able to agree what the relevant criteria are for establishing evidence of pain.

One problem, common to all moral principles and their supporting theories if we attempt to use them to resolve moral disagreement, is that since they are the source of the dispute, i.e. disputes would not arise in the first place if there were no conflicting moral principles, then it may not be very illuminating to appeal to them as a means of resolution. A utilitarian who derives a particular moral judgement about an action from the principle of utility cannot represent this process as offering a justification for the judgement he derives, for then the reason he is presenting to an opponent for the moral supremacy of his choice of action is nothing more than the reason for his making the choice in the first place. It is precisely because his opponent rejects this reasoning that the disagreement has occurred. Disputes between utilitarians are clearly not subject to this difficulty. If utilitarian theory is to be internally consistent, disputes must be resolvable even if, for reasons shown earlier, this is practically difficult. If two utilitarians held opposing beliefs about what to do in the first example of the man on the ventilator, then resolution should be possible if one party is able to convince the other that he has not done his calculations of utility correctly.

When we consider the sort of dispute that may arise between a utilitarian and a non-utilitarian the situation seems even more complex. I shall take as an example the dispute between a research scientist and the animal liberation group, as discussed in a recent

Guardian article by Polly Toynbee.[5] The doctor concerned, who is victim of a harassment campaign, is working on new drugs to combat epilepsy. He uses baboons to test the efficacy of the drugs, by first inducing fits by subjecting the baboons to a stroboscope, then injecting the drug and finally subjecting the baboons to the stroboscope again to see whether the drug has successfully inhibited their tendency to have fits. Toynbee concludes the article by saying that we have to choose between 'the use of baboons or the life and happiness of humans', and it is clear that the article is not an unbiased report but an article supporting the research on utilitarian grounds. Letters were later published from supporters of both sides in the dispute. It may be helpful to examine some of the arguments expressed and try to assess whether any of them might be useful for resolving the dispute.

Toynbee argues that although the baboons 'probably' do suffer, '100,000 human epileptics suffer horribly, year after year, living restricted and miserable lives, in constant fear of the terrible damage they do to themselves when they fall violently to the ground' and the 'good to human beings outweighs the harm to animals'. She is also concerned to minimise her assessment of the harm that the baboons suffer, arguing that this arises more from their experience of captivity than the experiments themselves and that the fits induced are mild, and the monkeys 'sit quite calmly' when strapped into their chairs. She seems to be making the sort of utilitarian calculation required by the 1876 Cruelty to Animals Act. To comply with this Act experimenters were required to state the net gain expected from the experiment and the net loss to the animals involved. Thus, she argues that the research is justified because it results in greater happiness than if it were not carried out. A supporting letter, from the husband of a deceased epileptic, goes further, stating that in order to prevent others from going through the 'hell' his wife experienced, he would 'personally perform any experiment on thousands of monkeys'. For this letter writer the research is justified by its human benefits without any consideration for the monkeys' suffering.

It would be wrong to present this debate simply in terms of a utilitarian/non-utilitarian conflict. Indeed one reader argued against the research on the grounds that vivisection may be detrimental to human health and it can lead to the use of drugs which are ineffective or dangerous, since baboons are inappropriate models for testing. However most arguments against the research emphasised that there is no moral justification for trying to cure human disease by inflicting disease and death on animals; it can never be right to inflict pain and suffering on a sentient creature for someone else's benefit.

How might the dispute be resolved? The possible reasons that can be offered appear limited. Resolution might be achieved if it could be shown that the research does not achieve the ends that it claims – the inappropriate model argument – or that there are available techniques for achieving experimental results which do not rely on baboons. Both parties could also use variants of the recognised method of moral argument, 'How would you like it if somebody did this to you', e.g. how would you feel if you were the unfortunate monkey/epileptic? It is, perhaps significant that both these arguments are not utilitarian.

The utilitarian seems to be reduced to continuing to point out the human benefits of the research. *If* his opponent had not known about these when he made his judgement, then he might possibly alter his views, but surely the whole basis of this dispute is that the Animal Rights supporter does already know and rejects their having any moral significance. The AR supporter is claiming that the research is immoral at the time of its inception; its consequences, however valuable, cannot make it moral.

Each party is arguing from within their own moral framework – they 'see different worlds'. People involved in animal rights issues question the whole moral attitude the research scientist displays towards the world. They claim we should share our planet with animals and not assume dominion over it. Resolution might occur if one party simply 'comes to see' that the other party is right. No doubt such conversions do sometimes happen and one party comes to adopt the other's moral framework, but more commonly the dispute ends in radical moral disagreement. Thus the use of utilitarian criteria will not resolve or even advance the debate, and although it is not the case that the utilitarian has nothing more to say he may have to accept there is nothing to be gained by saying it.

I conclude that: (1) Although a consideration of consequences is helpful in making a moral *decision* about an action, the morality of the action itself must also be subject to moral scrutiny in a way that the application of utilitarian criteria, by its very nature, ignores; (2) In attempting to resolve a dispute, utilitarian criteria are only useful if the other party has never even considered the consequences of the action he proposes. If he has and rejects their significance, then any expectation of the 'usefulness' of utilitarian criteria is misplaced; (3) In cases of radical moral disagreement where there appears to be no common evidence by which the dispute may be resolved, although we cannot say the dispute will never be resolved, it does not make sense to say there must be a solution. To this extent an appeal to utilitarian criteria may be just as 'useless' as any alternative strategy.

Notes

1. J. S. Mill, *Utilitarianism* (Everyman Edition) p. 6.
2. T. L Beauchamp and J. F. Childress, *Principles of Biomedical Ethics* (Oxford: Oxford University Press, 1983).
3. I. Kennedy, *The Unmasking of Medicine* (London: George Allen and Unwin, 1981). The case of Strunk *v* Strunk, p. 149.
4. J. L. Stocks, *Morality and Purposes* (London: Routledge & Kegan Paul, 1969).
5. P. Toynbee, 'Who's Torturing Whom?', *The Guardian*, October 1985.

6 The Status of the Foetus

Naomi Gilchrist

Arguments concerning the status of the foetus are not simply modern ones arising out of the increasing ability of medical science to manipulate the components of future and existing people. They have also arisen from the age-old problem of pregnancies that are for one reason or another undesirable. Consequently there exists a considerable body of opinion in society giving rise to much argument when moral dilemmas arise. These arguments are rooted in the problems of defining what is a human being, whether or not there is a moral distinction between a human being and a human person and also in questions of human rights. The results of such unresolved argument are evident in the inconsistent and ambiguous attitudes of society towards the foetus.

This essay will explore these areas in an attempt to show that, just as the status of human beings in society is an ethical consideration so too is the status of the human foetus. If this is the case, then it may follow that the foetus should be accorded the same rights as the rest of us, certainly in respect of its protection and survival. The most overt problems are likely to occur when legislation on certain points becomes necessary. British law must apply to everyone living under its jurisdiction and consequently serious difficulties may arise because of differing moral opinion. It is therefore necessary to consider the implications different moral stances may have for the formulation of laws. This will be followed by an account of how these matters affect my view of the issues discussed by the Warnock Committee.

While the terms embryo and zygote are used, for the purposes of this essay the term foetus may be taken to refer to the developing being from conception to birth. The foetus comes into existence as a result of human behaviour or action, i.e. because of sexual intercourse between two people or the co-operation of two such people with members of an institution such as the infertility clinic of a hospital. Glover[1] states that the foetus is an undoubted member of the human species and no one would dispute this. What is in dispute is whether or not the foetus should have the same right to life and the protection of the same that we all believe we should have. That is, is the foetus on equal terms with the rest of society when its life is in the balance? Should the protection of the foetus be a moral obligation on all of us? Opinions on this are very varied but I shall attempt to show that it should.

Ethics is concerned with the study of the principles and concepts by which human moral behaviour may be assessed or judged, possibly in a particular field such as medical science but also in communities or societies of people. If the foetus is a member of the human species and its existence is brought about by human behaviour then it follows that its existence and consequently any act that caused this existence to be terminated should also be the concern of ethics. However, attempts have been made to show that the foetus at certain stages of its development need not have ethical status and some of these will be examined below.

Status is a term relating to a position or rank in society and so, by definition, something conferred as a result of existence within such a group. Status has implicit value because decisions regarding status involve value judgements and also rights and obligations. It is usually conferred as a result of some kind of utility value to society. Consequently the giving of status involves judgements that are part of a given value system, i.e. part of morality.

Foetal status is conferred by the particular group into which the child would eventually be born. It follows that foetal status might be variable in our society because of different belief systems tending to generate different moral codes. If one considers those arising from major religions such as Christianity, Islam, Hinduism and all their variants, together with secular and humanist views, it is clear that moral consensus would be unlikely on important issues, such as this. Therefore the fact that the status of the foetus seems to be an ethical consideration does not solve but on the contrary generates the problem and arguments that arise when its survival is threatened in some way. Some seek to reduce the status of the foetus to the lowest possible level, that of human tissue, compared to other body tissues which may be disposed of or possibly exchanged if inconvenient or pathological. Unwanted pregnancy or an abnormal foetus might be placed almost in the category of disease for people of this persuasion. It would be consistent with this view not to attach any special significance to the foetus at all, thus arguing that foetal status need not be an ethical consideration. Those who hold that a woman should have the sole right to decide what happens to her own body, and the foetus which is simply part of that body, would need to hold a view similar to this one in order for the foetus to be a disposable item.

Dee Wells[2] believes that 'human life begins at birth . . . that human life begins at the moment of conception is a religious tenet that makes no claim whatsoever to scientific truth'. This is simply a statement of opinion which can make no claim of its own to scientific truth! This whole area is prone to emotive inconsistency and ambiguous definition.

In the interest of clarification it is necessary to examine some points on the continuum of human development in an attempt to discover whether or not any one of them has particular significance or might possibly be used as evidence on which to base a judgement that the foetus might be accorded the same status and consequent protection as the rest of us.

Most sexually mature humans produce ova or sperm according to their gender and regular and natural waste of both these forms of human tissue occurs unless ova and sperm meet and fertilisation takes place. It is, therefore, difficult to attach any ethical significance to ova and sperm separately. Those mentioned above who argue that the foetus is simply human tissue claim that there is no real distinction between gametes and zygotes, i.e. that they are both live human tissue. However it seems difficult to discount the fact that all the necessary genetic material to make a new human being is now present and ready for development. Members of the Roman Catholic Church and those others who hold the 'sanctity of life'view believe that this new life, however rudimentary, should be protected as sacred and that no interference detrimental to its welfare should be allowed unless the life of the mother herself is threatened. This point brings into question the absolute nature of this view. If the mother's life is somehow more valuable than that of the foetus when only one of them can live, how can they then argue for equal status, i.e. no qualitative difference, if the question of foetal survival is raised on grounds other than those of saving maternal life? This is another instance of inconsistency in views on this subject.

After conception, implantation in the wall of the uterus is essential if the embryo is to go on developing. A considerable number of zygotes do not implant successfully and are shed in natural wastage unknown to anyone. This point is sometimes used in arguments against the view that conception is the most significant point, the time at which the development of a new human life begins. However implantation is concerned with the fulfilment of conditions necessary for survival and development once all genetic material is present; it is not concerned with the intrinsic value of the zygote itself. Moreover implantation is only necessary to the survival of the foetus at present: it is possible to foresee survival entirely outside the human body as medical science progresses. If it becomes possible at some future time to dispense with the human body as a foetal support system then it is no longer an essential condition and the notion of implantation as significant collapses. The significance of such necessary conditions for foetal survival and consequent fulfilment of potential will be expanded further below.

The development of the primitive streak, on the embryonic disc on the 14th or 15th day of development, is sometimes used in arguments against conception as a firm boundary because until this is established it is not known whether the embryo will develop into one person or two as in the case of monozygotic twins. 'But this objection is not fatal to the case for conception as the boundary.'[3] The fact that the embryo can become one person is sufficient to accord it protection and this 'possible twinning' argument simply begs the question and cannot justify interference with an embryo or reduce the significance of conception.

The importance of a nervous system enabling the foetus to feel pain is sometimes used in arguments to justify research on embryos before this point. Is research permissible if carried out before the foetus is developmentally able to feel pain? Again this is begging the question. Suffering would certainly be a consideration if and only if it had already been established that the foetus should not be accorded the protection due to human persons in general.

Quickening, the first detectable sign of foetal movement by the mother, was regarded by 'Augustine of Hippo and several other authorities . . . as a positive sign of ensoulment'.[4] Whatever the various beliefs have been on this point, it is hard to see what moral significance can be drawn from it today. Our modern understanding of the uninterrupted nature of foetal development from conception to birth removes any significance this may have had. It is also well known that an experienced mother feels her child move earlier in second and subsequent pregnancies, which introduces an element of arbitrariness into the fixing of this pleasant event in time. It is of emotional significance for the mother, not of moral significance for the status of the foetus.

After the 28th week of gestation the foetus is considered legally viable. This point draws a useful legal line when a birth is not a live one, namely that between stillbirth and miscarriage. This was thought to be the earliest possible time when the foetus, if born, might survive. The attraction of viability as a significant point in foetal development is that the possibility for live independence is real for the first time since conception. The problem lies not only in the idea, which again is about necessary conditions, but also in the 28 weeks attached to it. Already the medical recommendations are for pushing back viability to 24 weeks of gestation. Singer[5] has pointed out that 'a six-month-old foetus might have a fair chance of survival if born in a city like London or New York where the latest medical techniques are used but no chance at all if born in a remote village in Chad or New Guinea'.

Viability it seems has a legal but not a moral significance, it is a 'moveable feast' which is of no help when trying to establish the status of the foetus other than when it is born dead before full term. Midwives are known to attempt resuscitation on foetuses which miscarry before this time but show signs of life, indicating that 28 weeks holds no real moral significance to them in terms of whether the foetus lives or dies.

The last point to be considered is birth itself, again a 'moveable feast' in the light of what has been said about viability. What could possibly count as evidence that the status of the foetus of 39 weeks gestation is a different moral consideration from that of a full-term neonate? And what of the comparison between a foetus of 39 weeks and a premature neonate of 36 weeks gestation? Both the foetus and the neonate can hear and feel their mother's body. The difference between them is minimal and physiological and not one on which moral distinctions can be founded.

Apart from conception, when all the genetic material for the creation of a new person is present, this examination has failed to establish any significant point on the continuum of foetal development at which there is a qualitative change in the foetus sufficient to enable it to stand as evidence for a change of status. Any status accorded to the foetus must therefore be present from conception onwards through into life after birth. At all stages of development the foetus and also the neonate need suitable conditions in order to survive. Remove these from the neonate and it will die as will the zygote that fails to implant. If the removal of such conditions from the neonate is unethical then it follows that it is so to remove them from the foetus. Therefore the foetus, from conception onwards, should be regarded as a human person and granted the same status in all matters concerning its protection from harm and consequently its ultimate survival.

A view in opposition to this, and one that might be used to support abortion or embryo research, is that although the foetus may be regarded as a human being it is not yet a human person and consequently not due to the rights and protection to which people are due. This is a question of definition, that is what one understands by the words 'human being' and 'human person'. Michael Tooley[6] equates personhood with being a bearer of rights, and argues that a bearer of rights 'must have at least the capacity to desire what they have a right to'. Tooley's conclusion is that as the foetus can desire nothing, as far as we know, then it follows that it has no rights.

Referring to the point made above that the existence of the foetus is generally caused by informed human behaviour, I would take issue with Tooley and argue that such behaviour incurs an obligation, on the part of its creators, towards the foetus. It would seem irresponsible and contradictory to create a human life and then to seek to destroy it. Anyone who acts to create a human life has, therefore, an obligation towards that life, and an obligation to protect it. This appears to invest the foetus with a right to life based on the 'doctrine of the "logical correlativity" of obligations and rights, a right entails that someone else has an obligation to act in certain ways'.[7]

This doctrine of logical correlativity works in both directions, i.e. that obligations entail rights and that rights entail obligations. Nevertheless there remains a distinction between the foetus and a person. Becoming a person is the result of living in the world, being conscious, interacting with other people and developing the ability for rational thought and moral behaviour. Such experience creates a recognisably individual personality with notions of rights and obligation. Tooley's assumption is that such a person is more valuable than the 'tabula rasa' that is, the foetus or neonate. My contention is that to place more intrinsic value on a person because he or she has had more time and experience is no basis for a valid argument. It is the equivalent of saying that a child of five years is less valuable than one of ten years. Personhood develops slowly, it does not simply happen in a day or two. There is a distinction between these two but not one of moral value, simply one of experience and expertise. Time, if allowed to pass, will reduce any such difference until it ceases to exist and consequently absence of awareness of rights or anything else cannot be used as a basis for value judgements on foetal worth.

Consider those 'feral' children raised outside human society. The Indian girl Amala appeared to have no notion of rights or any idea of human behaviour or language. This was not considered to be a reason for letting her die or killing her; on the contrary, she was cared for with love and patience by the people to whom she was taken. Mentally subnormal people may have very little awareness or no notion of their rights, but our society does not prescribe euthanasia for them on these grounds.

That the foetus, feral children and the mentally handicapped have not developed such awareness is due to problems of incomplete development for reasons such as lack of time, wrong circumstances or physical damage. Normal healthy neonates have much developing to do before they acquire the awareness and capacities to which Tooley refers and yet they are awarded the rights and protection that all of us hope for from the society in which we live. How then can the foetus be denied such rights if, as has been demonstrated, a point cannot be fixed between conception and the dawning awareness of personhood in early childhood which would indicate a change in the foetus or neonate significant enough to alter its status?

However, the disputes still remain because different groups of people confer different value on the foetus. This was clear in the expressions of dissent within the Warnock Report and is regularly expressed in arguments about abortion. This is not surprising: we live in a pluralist society with many different groups which can be defined according to their different beliefs. It follow that there will be disagreement between such groups on important questions such as the purpose of life, the existence of God, the definition of a human being or person, and possibly whether or not the foetus is one, both or neither of these things. W. D. Hudson[8] explores the possibility that as different ideologies have different views of man so different moral systems evolve in order to support man in achieving the ideal of his particular world view. Hudson (1970, p. 321) states: 'There does seem to be some connection between anthropology and ethics, that is, between what it is believed a man is and what it is believed that he ought to do.'

Hudson goes on to use examples of ideologies in opposition to one another such as those of existentialists and religious moralists. There are many others. He bases these views on the notion of human flourishing, i.e. that moral systems evolve to nurture a particular theory of human nature, and he goes on to demand consistency between one's view of man and one's morality. A belief system such as Catholicism demonstrates such consistency, teaching that God, having endowed the foetus with a soul, forbids any interference damaging to foetal welfare. The Roman Catholic Church accords the foetus the protection accorded to everyone. The view that the foetus is simply human tissue would only be consistent if it is held to be true for all foetuses during the whole gestation period. It cannot be true only for those ones that are unwanted, damaged or the product of rape. Most women who are expecting a wanted baby regard it very differently from the way in which they might regard their appendix, for example.

Society recognises the freedom of different groups to hold different beliefs, and so it follows that society must recognise that different sets of moral rules have a valid contribution to make in the determination of the content of belief regarding what is and what ought to be the case. If relativism rules and it is accepted that there is no ethical absolute that all groups can come to accept, could there be any other standard that might be found to be mutually acceptable? One thing that all groups have in common is their humanity. Perhaps Hudson's notion of human flourishing could be applied at this fundamental level. Perhaps there are ethical decisions that in their reference to our humanity depend on human sentiment for their justification, such as, who would deny that children should not go hungry or that aid should be given to people rendered injured or helpless by an accident? There appears to be an area of human common sense and compassion where what is to be done is evident, but not objectively so, in terms of our common humanity. The problem with this humane reasoning arises when choices have to be made. Suppose the Good Samaritan had been on a life-saving mission with only enough time and resources to save or obtain help for a person in his home? How does he choose between that one and the man set upon by thieves? It seems that we are forced back upon 'the lesser of two evils' and a general utilitarian judgement for the maximisation of happiness and good health. Such reasoning was evident in the Abortion Act.

In view of what has been said on the plurality of respected moral views it would seem impossible to uphold all of these when formulating or advising on a law to regulate and control measures concerning human fertilisation and embryology. However, what evidence is there to support the view that law should enforce morality or even the view of the majority on a particular moral problem? This seems to be a popular misconception. The law that absolutely prohibited abortion in the UK probably upheld the majority view of the day that abortion was morally wrong. Peter Singer[9] argues that this law drove abortion underground, producing many bad effects; he quotes the Canadian Royal Commission (on the status of women) which opposed these laws: 'A law that has more bad effects than good ones is a bad law . . .' This is a utilitarian judgement which recognises that abortion was happening in spite of the law and is in favour of controlled abortion under laid down conditions or circumstances. This was intended to reduce the bad consequences of back street, illegal abortion and make it safe by allowing safer medical termination of pregnancy. In this instance it seems that a law, contrary to the majority of moral opinion of the time would have been a better law.

Another instance where it is possible to demonstrate utilitarian justification of a law which opposes morality is in the statutory provision of armed forces in opposition to the moral law prohibiting killing. Many sections of our forces are trained as effective killing machines but, in this country, are generally assumed to be for use in defence of the realm and our democratic way of life; the justification for killing in war is to prevent the bad consequences that would occur if these were overthrown. That these institutions have the support and co-operation of the Anglican and Roman Catholic Churches is curious and significant, for not many exceptions are made to the law of the Ten Commandments: it must mean, therefore, that in the Church's view the law need not always be restricted to enforce aspects of morality if a greater good can be envisaged by transgression of the same.

A good law, then, is one that produces more benefits than harms for society when all aspects surrounding its effect have been taken into account. However, when such a law is in conflict with morality, stringent controls are necessary in order to exert sufficient control to prevent abuse of this apparent dispensation to behave contrary to morality. Consider, for example, the criteria necessary to justify carrying out abortion in present-day Britain.

The Warnock Report examines all the techniques involved in fertility treatment and embryo research and their surrounding issues carefully and humanely, and has drawn up a system of controls and regulations in Chapter 13.[10] The problem for the Committee was how to get to the point where this could be done. The purpose of the report was to make recommendations which might lead to legislation. It is important not to lose sight of this point because, as we have seen above, laws must apply to everyone regardless of their particular moral viewpoint. The Committee did not arrive at a consensus on issues such as some aspects of surrogacy, and embryo research. Lady Warnock was obviously aware of this possibility at the outset and quoted David Hume, who wrote that morality 'was more properly felt than judg'd of'.[11] Lady Warnock admitted the necessity of recourse to moral sentiment because 'neither utilitarianism nor blind obedience to rules could solve the moral dilemmas the inquiry was faced with' – that is, that most of the techniques investigated do harm human embryos and are consequently morally offensive to a great many people, some of whom were on the Committee. But there is a problem with 'moral feeling': if I feel one thing is right and you feel another thing is right and mine wrong, how would anyone judge between our two views? How does one come to 'feel' that something is morally wrong? In some way we must have internalised principles and information that enable us to make such judgements either from existing moral codes or simply from being part of the human race. Beauchamp and Walters[12] put forward some arguments against cultural relativism: 'Among the best known are arguments that there is a universal structure of human nature or at least a universal set of human needs which leads to the adoption of similar or even identical principles in our cultures.'

It could be that shared human experience will show a shared moral feeling if analysed back into fundamental principles. However, no attempt was made to examine opposing moral views in the Report, and this appeal to moral sentiment appears to have little use or effect other than to allay public fears that moral feeling was about to be outraged.

The Report is remarkable for its clarity of language and argument. However it is my contention that this clarity and the appeal to moral sentiment tend to hide the fact that the recommendations of the Inquiry, despite Lady Warnock's claims, are really simply utilitarian ones. She states: 'For that a decision is based on sentiment by no means entails that arguments cannot be adduced to support it. Nor are utilitarian arguments based on possible benefits and harms ruled out. It is only that they will not suffice alone.'[13] But in the end they do seem to suffice alone. The document examines the possible benefits from the eradication or avoidance of genetic disorder, the happiness of people (a somewhat shaky utilitarian assessment), when they eventually become parents and acknowledges the harm to embryos. The moral feeling of those who disagree with harming embryos is set aside in expressions of dissent. It is however consistent with other permitted measures in our society, when killing people must be justified by such a benefit/harms calculus, and it is morally consistent with these other problematic areas.

If the findings of the Inquiry are supported by utilitarian arguments there is surely a weakness in the avoidance of any discussion about financial resources. The Report states that: 'While we accept that questions about the uses of resources are proper questions . . . - essentially they relate to the extent of provision, not to whether there should be any provision at all.'[14] In a 'benefits and harms' assessment how can one avoid taking into account living people who may not receive treatment soon enough or at all if money is spent creating more people in this way? There is an interesting tension between the creation of these much desired children and the resultant availability of embryos for research purposes. Is the alleviation of infertility carried out for its own sake in a genuine attempt to help infertile couples or might it be a product of mankind's hubris encouraged mainly because it provides the raw materials for embryo research? This aspect is not addressed by the Report and is perhaps a cynical view, but in the light of limited resources in the National Health Service one that it is difficult to ignore.

One is left with the uneasy feeling that the Warnock Report has ingeniously papered over some cracks in order to allow research in this area to continue, and was about sensitive assessment of necessary controls rather than an attempt to provide a moral justification for the techniques under examination which would be of assistance in the formulation of laws.

Notes

1. J. Glover, *Causing Death and Saving Lives* (Harmondsworth: Pelican, 1977) p. 121.
2. Dee Wells, *The Guardian*, 29 November 1973, reprinted in Glover, op. cit., p. 119.
3. J. Glover, op. cit., p. 123.
4. A. V. Campbell, *Moral Dilemmas in Medicine* (Churchill Livingstone, 1972) p. 124.

5. P. Singer, *Practical Ethics* (Oxford: Oxford University Press, 1979) p. 109.
6. M. Tooley, 'Abortion and Infanticide' (*Philosophy and Public Affairs*, 1972), quoted in Glover, op. cit., p. 127.
7. T. L. Beauchamp and J. F. Childress, *Principles of Biomedical Ethics* (Oxford: Oxford University Press, 1983) p. 512.
8. W. D. Hudson, *Modern Moral Philosophy* (London: Macmillan, 1970) p. 321
9. P. Singer, op. cit., p. 111.
10. M. Warnock, *A Question of Life* (Oxford: Blackwell, 1985).
11. M. Warnock, op. cit., pp. viii–ix.
12. Beauchamp and Walters (eds), *Contemporary Issues in Bioethics* (Belmont: Wadsworth, 1982) p. 8.
13. M. Warnock, op. cit., p. x.
14. M. Warnock, op. cit., pp. 32, 58.

7 Should my Baby Live?

Sylvia Parker

It was 2.30 a.m. My baby son had been born exactly twenty-four hours earlier, and my wakefulness should have been for the purpose of feeding and caring for him. Instead, I lay exhausted, trying to come to terms with the awful reality that I was now the mother of a grossly handicapped child. Presently I must have slept, for I found myself walking alone into a conference room. In the centre was an oblong table, and seated along either side, were a number of people whom I recognised as eminent philosophers. I took a seat at one end, leaving the chair at the head of the table vacant. The doctor in charge of my son's case was also present, and it was he who commenced the proceedings. Briefly, he explained to the assembled group, that my son had been born with a serious spinal lesion which would result in permanent physical and mental handicap, and that I, as his parent, was required to authorise medical treatment without which he would eventually die.

'The purpose of this conference,' he continued, 'is to provide Sylvia with philosophical concepts from each of your perspectives in such a way as to clarify the morality of the decision she now faces. The question is, "Should her baby live, or should he die?"'.

In turn, those around the table then began to speak. Epicurus was first: 'It is my belief', he said, 'that our human existence is simply a diminutive part of a universal whole. Every event is the result, or reaction of the energy of atoms as they indeterminately move in different directions through time and space. The occurrence of human life is the natural consequence of a conglomerate of past events.

I do not accept the theory that God is a separate entity and the creator of all things. My beliefs are Pantheistic. God is nature, and nature is God. It is natural for man to love nature, since it is a part of his own existence. It is, likewise, natural for man to love God for the same reason, but as it would be ludicrous to expect nature to love him in return, so it would be unreasonable to expect God to love and care for him.

I suggest, that because you cannot change your circumstances or future events, and cannot therefore be held morally responsible for these, that you choose a line of action which will cause you the least amount of pain. It is our moral duty as human beings to learn acceptance of all the events in our lives, to avoid struggling against the inevitable and to seek the greatest happiness in any given set of circumstances.

If your baby is allowed to die or is killed now, you are bound to suffer extreme anguish, and the pain is likely to remain with you, and change to some extent your whole outlook on the rest of your life. You will, though, be spared the trauma of watching his grotesque little body grow abnormally to become more and more unacceptable to society; and worse, to wonder when he makes those inevitable inhuman sounds, whether he is suffering inestimable agony.

Your approach in this should be a Hedonistic one; seek to do that which will in the long term give you most pleasure.'

Spinoza was the next to speak: 'This painful event in your life,' he said, 'is only good or bad in as much as your own mind is affected by it. Good and bad are relative concepts, and to have borne a physically and mentally handicapped child is good or bad only to the extent to which you allow the occurrence to affect the way you feel. In other words, it is your own emotions, your own perception of your son and his disabilities which determine whether this event in your life is good or bad. There are no perfect children. Perfection, like beauty, is in the eye of the beholder. Your son is what you perceive him to be, and what you choose for him will be decided by your concept of him.

I believe that the ordinary surroundings of life which are esteemed by men to be the highest good, may be classed under three headings: Riches, Fame and Pleasure of sense. With these three, the mind is so absorbed that it has little power to reflect on any different good.

This experience in your life may be your salvation, for by turning away from your natural search for riches, fame or sensual pleasure, all of which are perishable, you free your mind to search for the hidden joy and happiness of life.'

Spinoza thus concluded his discourse and Bentham began.

'I hold Utilitarian beliefs,' he explained, 'and am a Consequentialist. I think that an action is right or wrong in so far as it tends to produce the greatest happiness for the greatest number.

If you calculate the good consequences of allowing your son to live against the bad consequences, you will be able to determine the rightness or wrongness of your decision.

The choice you make for your son will determine not only all the good or evil which will befall him, but also all the good or evil which will be experienced by others, such as members of your family, friends and carers. If you choose life for your son, you must ask yourself who will care for him and how will such care be financed. If you choose his death, how will it affect those around you, and who will actually do the killing. You may decide that to kill your child is a moral act for you, but you are then faced with the question of whether you would have to accept the responsibility for having set a precedent for other parents in similar circumstances who may adopt your values without much thought as to whether the same decision would be appropriate for them.

For whose benefit do you decide? If you choose life for your son, will the purpose of that choice be for the gratification of your own maternal needs or from a genuine altruistic wish to protect his right to life? If you choose the latter, you must determine the worth of the life you are preserving. To whom will such a life be of value? What is it that makes a life worthwhile? Is it the ability to think, to use one's mind? Does the act of thinking exist independently of the ability to communicate ideas? If so, is an active mind trapped within a body totally incapable of transmitting those thoughts of any value?

Is it a good thing, or a bad thing, to preserve lives which have no value?'

Kant then made the next contribution.

'Every person's life is an end in itself, and not merely a means to an end. It would be wrong, therefore, assuming that you believe your son to be a person with equal human rights, to deny him his life. A just society is one in which each individual, no matter what his station in life, is treated equally before the law, and is the subject of equal concern by society. To be moral we must be fair.

I say, that it is not the consequences of the decision you make, but your motive for your action which is morally significant. In coming to your decision you must suppress your own desires and act from a sense of obligation. If you make your decision believing it to be a moral one, then even if the consequences are bad, the act itself will have been a right one.

Remember too, that every action must be judged in the light of how it would appear if it were to be a universal code of behaviour. You cannot decide that to kill your son is a moral action, unless you agree that it would be right to kill all grossly handicapped infants. It is your duty to ensure that your decision is made for the right reasons'.

Ross put in a sentence here. He said 'You should make your decision in the knowledge that it is not your motive, nor yet the consequences of the act, but the morality of the act itself which counts. Is the act of maintaining your son's life a right one, or is the act of killing him a right one? I say that our morality is judged by the rightness or wrongness of the act itself.'

Ayn Rand was the only female philosopher present, and her theory was perhaps harder to accept than any of the others.

'I shall deal with your problem by looking briefly at the issue of man's rights,' she stated. 'A right is a moral principle defining and sanctioning a man's freedom of action in a social context. There is only one fundamental right – a man's right to his own life. The right to life means the right to engage in self sustaining and self generated action, which means: the freedom to take all the actions required by the nature of a rational being for the support, the furtherance, the fulfillment and the enjoyment of his own life.

Our western society in its efforts to encourage altruism at the expense of a healthy egoism, may have led you to believe that individuals like your son have a right to life, but I ask, at whose expense? He, like all others unable to provide for themselves, place a huge financial and emotional burden upon society, and any alleged right of one man which necessitates the violation of the rights of another is not, and cannot be a right. A man has a right to life only if he can support himself: if he cannot, others who support him become his slaves.'

After a long pause, St Paul, adopting a very broad perspective, expounded the christian ethic.

'God is good', he began, 'God is the supreme and immortal creator of all things. He is omniscient, omnipotent and omnipresent, and nothing happens unless He wills it. Morality and God are synonymous. God does not strive to uphold moral principles, but is superior to them. Significant to our discussion today are the concepts of sin, and of life after death. The man who fails to acknowledge God as Lord, forsakes the good, and thereby condemns himself to eternal Hell, or separation from the good, but the man who recognises his sinful state and asks forgiveness, is sanctified, and rewarded with eternal life after death.

Whether man has any choice in the matter, has been debated for centuries. The opposite poles of Determinism and Liberalism, from both a religious and a scientific point of view, remain a subject for much speculation.

Determinists claim that every action of every human being is predestined, so that nothing we can ever do can alter the ultimate outcome of our lives. Liberalists, on the other hand, believe that we are free to make our own choices and thereby determine our own destinies.

The birth of your handicapped son is not without purpose, "For all things work together for good to them that love God", but the christian ethic is not clear about the fate of those who die in ignorance of the christian faith. The scriptures tell us that "We are born in sin and shapen in iniquity", and that "All have sinned and come short of the glory of God", thus condemning us all to eternal damnation.

On the other hand, Jesus said, "Suffer little children to come unto me, – for of such is the kingdom of Heaven".

One of your chief considerations when choosing life or death for your son must be the lawfulness of your action. God commanded Moses to write on tablets of stone "Thou shalt not kill". Your laws today firmly uphold that ancient rule, so in authorising your son's killing you will have broken both God's commandment, and your current societal law.'

Having completed their discourse, each of my advisors turned to face me, and overwhelmed by the burden which weighed so heavily upon me, I sat for some time with eyes closed. When at last I opened them, it was to find that the chair facing me at the head of the table, was now occupied by a mystical being whom I recognised as my son. He nodded affectionately, and directing his comments towards me, said, 'I know that you love me Mother. You feel the biological and emotional ties between us which are natural following any normal human birth, and yet you look at my deformed little body in the incubator and wonder what went wrong, and why this awful thing has happened to us. You remember the lively healthy children born to others around you, and also some of the grossly abnormal ones.

There was one in particular; a child with hydrocephalus, whom you as a midwife delivered back in 1970. Do you remember? After only a few days her head began to grow disproportionately to the rest of her body. Week after week she clung tenaciously to life until the stretched skin shone, and the tense blue blood vessels pulsed as though they would burst at any moment. At ten weeks old the tiny child needed two nurses to turn her; one to hold her body, the other to hold her head, now so huge and heavy, that care had to be taken that her neck was not broken in the process. She had to be lowered into her cot in such a way as to ensure that her head would fit between the sides of the cot. Both her ears and the surrounding areas were badly excoriated, bleeding and infected.

Day after day, grim faced doctors and nurses doggedly continued to feed and care for her, trying to ignore her pathetic whimpering, and fervently wishing that she would die.

Remember also, the mother who once told you that caring for her severely handicapped child had been the most rewarding experience of her life: that the child's existence had enriched her own life, and given her a sense of purpose and fulfillment far greater than any other event in her life had afforded.

I am not able to help you with the decision you now have to make concerning my future; I simply exist in the form of a helpless deformed little body. You cannot know if I am aware of myself, or of that which exists outside of myself. You cannot know if I feel pain, or simply react instinctively to internal and/or external stimuli; for to experience pain, or any other sensation I must have some degree of awareness.

So now you must reach a decision. You have but two options for me – life or death. But before you decide, there are many questions you must ask yourself.

Has my life the same worth as other lives? Is the value of a life measured by some fixed moral standard? If so, what is that standard, and who sets it? Is my little inert body really a person, in the same sense that you are a person? What exactly are the qualities that constitute personhood? Ramsey would say that my life is a gift from God and is therefore sacred, and because of God's timeless quality, my short life of perhaps weeks or months is of the same value to Him, as the life which spans seventy-two years.

Will you approach this problem of yours in a hardheaded and practical way, as Rand would, and condemn me to death because I will never be in a position to support myself and thereby earn a right to my life? Will you deny me a comfortable death because the law forbids you to kill, or allow to die, another human being?

Will you follow Bentham's advice, and decide my future on utilitarian grounds, or will you appraise the acts of killing and of maintaining life for what they really are, and uphold one of these because it appears to be the most moral act of the two?'

There was a long pause. My mind began to contemplate even

more questions. Is there a ultimate purpose for the human race, I wondered, and if so, are we as individuals meant to participate in achieving that purpose? My weariness and confusion were greater than I could bear.

A midwife woke me with a cup of tea, and I remembered that I had a decision to make.

References

Kuhse, H. and Singer, P., *Should the Baby Live? Problems of Handicapped Infants* (Oxford: Oxford University Press, 1985)

Glover, J., *Causing Death and Saving Lives* (Harmondsworth: Penguin, 1977).

Rand, A., *The Virtue of Selfishness* (New York: New American Library, 1964).

Popkin, R. and Stroll, A., *Introduction to Philosophy* (New York: Holt, Rinehart and Winston, 1979).

Smart, J. J., and Williams, B., *Utilitarianism. For and Against* (Cambridge: Cambridge University Press, 1973).

The Bible, The Old and New Testaments: Romans 8: 28; Psalm 51: 5; Romans 3: 23; Matthew 19: 14; and Deut. 5: 17.

8 The Limits of Health Care

David Moore

'In the beginning, middle and end, was, is and will be scarcity of resources.'[1]

This essay starts from the premise that the demand for and possibilities of health-care provision will always be greater than the available resources. For the purpose of comparing the moral significance of cost-benefit and cost-effectiveness analyses, the debate as to whether an allocation of 6.2 per cent (1983) of Great Britain's gross national product to health care can be justified against allocations to defence, education and other public services, is assumed to be unproblematic.[2] The economists' simple truth that demand will always outstrip resources is taken as an a priori assumption. The inevitable consequence of this assumption is choice – choice as to which health-care programmes should be pursued and to what extent.

The apparently insatiable appetite of health-care consumers and the finite resources available have resulted in decisions being made by default, without reasoned judgement and in response to 'decibel pressure'.[3] The same author continues that 'it is time, we as a nation, were more rational in setting priorities'.[4] The reasoned judgement and rationality appealed for seems to have entered the arena in the form of health economics. In particular two techniques of economic evaluation have been elaborated[5] and widely reviewed and espoused.[6] Economic appraisal as a means of assisting in health-care spending allocation decisions has utilised the techniques of cost-benefit analysis (CBA) and cost-effectiveness analysis (CEA). The two techniques are, on the surface, remarkably similar in the sense that both require the detailed analysis of both costs and benefits of health-care interventions. It has been stressed in the literature that such analyses should take into account all costs and benefits regardless upon whom they fall.[7] Such analyses are therefore unlikely to be restricted only to health service inputs and outputs. Indeed, in referring to the work of Sugden and Williams,

Copp makes the point that the standard approach requires 'all of the costs and benefits of a project, to all the individual members of the relevant society, . . . to be taken into account, discounting future costs and benefits, ideally at the rate of time preference of each person concerned'.[8] The purpose of such a rigorous analysis is to assist decision makers in pursuit of the most efficient options in health-care provision. Efficiency is at the heart of both CBA and CEA since, as Maynard has pointed out, the economists' position is that 'inefficiency is unethical'.[9] Mooney too argues that 'the ethic is that of the common good and, indeed, not settling for doing good but doing better, more fairly'.[10] Let us first consider the moral significance of cost-effectiveness analysis.

CEA is concerned with the relative efficiency of competing treatments or interventions in the achievement of a particular goal. This implies that the most rational choice or resource investment is the option which yields the greatest benefit for least cost. On the face of it this method of assisting in decisions about which option to invest in, to achieve an agreed health-care goal, is morally benign. It is difficult to argue that any decision maker would be ethically unjustified in seeking to maximise health-care provision by investing the least resources in a given programme to achieve a stated goal. Providing CEA is applied in a politically and morally neutral manner, that is to say, it is not used deliberately to discredit or devalue a particular approach to health care in order to assert pre-eminence of a predetermined political or moral position, then there can be little ethical objection to its application in the process of making decisions regarding health-care spending.

However, one significant potential flaw remains, that of the measurement and valuation of the costs and benefits of health care. The definition of health itself is highly contentious. Agreement is minimal and the widely quoted World Health Organisation's definition, 'physical, mental and social well-being, and not merely the absence of disease or infirmity', also presents problems of health measurement and valuation.[11] Given that there is little agreement on what it is that is being measured, the units of measurement and the relative weighting placed upon them can be little more than the value judgements that the technique seeks to overcome. Indeed Drummond, asserting the need to express all the relevant costs and benefits in commensurate units, admits that this may not always be practicable and either a more restricted question needs to be posed, or the decision maker must 'exercise more of his own judgement'.[12]

Muir Gray, in a critique of economic appraisal in choosing priorities goes further and argues that such choices have to be made on ethical not financial grounds.[13] It might be argued then that the facade of objectivity that CEA implies and economists claim, is little more than a disguise for one set of values in preference to another. The economist, unprepared to assert the rightness of his case in valuing a particular course of action in open ethical debate, conceals these values within a system of fallacious measures and subterfuge – CEA.

The moral objection to CEA should not be taken as an absolute denial of the usefulness of the technique. Indeed it may prove the most useful tool available to establish the relative merits of competing claims. Even Muir-Gray acknowledges that the most important criterion in choosing priorities should be the effectiveness of the service.[14] It may also be the most adequate response to decibel pressure (and in 'particular the medical lobby),[15] currently available but only to the extent to which, in its application, there is a readiness to admit to its limitations and the extent to which the valuation of health-care input and output measurement is no more than an implicit moral evaluation of their relative worth.

This latter criticism is especially applicable to instances where monetary valuation proves problematic and other means are used. The development of Quality Adjusted Life Years (pronounced Qually to rhyme with Wally, according to Harris!)[16] and other algorithmic health indices[17] is a good illustration of the tactic of objectifying and of making covert certain moral imperatives. In reality no patient experiences a quality adjusted life year but a degree of distress and or disability perceived accurately and measured against the value of their life as rated only by them. No theoretical statistical abstraction can truly hope to gauge accurately a judgement about the quality and value of the life of another. Recourse to statistical abstraction may lessen the burden of choice borne by health-care spending allocators but the apparent objectivity and consequential rightness claimed for the 'efficiency ethic', is little more than an unconscious denial or intellectualisation of the underlying moral implications of their actions, analogous perhaps to doctors' and nurses' denial of ethical dilemmas by reference to decisions as 'medical' or 'clinical'.

In summary then, the moral significance of CEA in health-care spending is relatively benign, given neutrality in its application together with an explicit acknowledgement of the extent to which it is no less value laden than any other process involving an evaluation of costs and benefits as applied to human life. This characterisation is in contrast to the potentially more malignant and pervasive application of CBA. Whereas CEA is concerned with how best to achieve a specified objective, CBA is concerned with whether a particular health-care goal is worthy of pursuit.

The similarity of the mechanisms of measurement and valuation in both CEA and CBA ensure that the criticisms outlined above apply equally to the latter as to the former. However, these arguments will now be extended and developed in relation to CBA.

Mooney has articulated the two principles of CBA as, 'where benefits exceed costs and do not do those things where costs exceed benefits'.[18] This 'simple truth' as Williams[19] asserts depends entirely on an anlysis of costs and benefits. The important distinction between CEA and CBA is that the latter uses this analysis, not to evaluate the relative efficiency of two or more approaches to achieving the same goal, but in decisions about which objectives should be pursued (allocative efficiency) and to what extent (marginal allocation efficiency).

There is little doubt that decision makers in the health-care resource allocation system at all levels face difficult choices. Should resources be 'channelled into renal services in the knowledge that without dialysis certain death will follow, the cost being £15,000 per person per year for perhaps ten years . . . or channelled into hip replacements whereby people who are housebound not only throw away their crutches but live, laugh and are relieved of the burden of coping with themselves and can once again be concerned with others at a cost of £1,925 per one-off operation?'[20] These up-to-date costings of current health-care choices illustrate the economists' claim that life can be valued in monetary terms. Not to invest in dialysis implies that a renal patient's life is valued at less than £15,000 per year. Investment in such programmes implies such a life is valued at, at least, £150,000 (given a ten-year life span on dialysis). Valuation of this type can be computed against a number of criteria. For example, the value of a man's life could be considered to be a function of the productive capacity which would be lost if he were to die resulting in a diminished gross national product which generates the funds for health care in the first place. But is a contribution to gross national product a realistic measure of benefit? The consumer-sovereignty approach borrowed from market economics proposes that health-care consumers are the only true judges of benefit. The difficulty here is that there are practical problems in asking everyone how much they would be prepared to pay to avoid certain death. Mooney, Russell and Weir (1980) have argued, however, that a more realistic question is not 'how much would an individual – plus relatives, friends, etc., – be willing to pay to avoid certain death, but rather how much would such a group be prepared to pay to reduce the individual's risk of death from say x to y where x and y are very much less than one (where one equals certain death)'.[21] Muir Gray asserts that having calculated the value of a man's life, the cost of life saving services can be compared with the benefits that will accrue if lives are saved.[22] The economics of this are elaborated by Mooney *et al.* as follows: 'If 10,000 individuals are prepared to pay £1 on average to reduce their risk from 2 in 10,000 to 1 in 10,000, then the "value of life" (since one life would be saved) would be £10,000'.[23]

Muir-Gray believes the considerations outlined above to be problematic, especially in relation to disability. He argues that the value of life cannot be expressed in monetary terms and that the comparison of competing claims for resources such as renal programmes and special care baby units has to be made on ethical not on financial grounds.

One of the primary moral objections to CBA is that the value of life cannot be expressed in monetary terms. Initially this view might derive from a psychological revulsion to the notion that a life is worth '£x's but there is, perhaps more importantly, moral justification in a refusal to value life in monetary terms.[24] Fried has made the point that 'the touchstone of value is persons – free persons, moral persons'.[25] This Kantian view claims that the source of value of persons is the capacity of persons to reflect, to reach judgements and to make judgements about truth and falsehood and how they should live their lives and treat others.

Harris makes the point that life saving has special importance because continued existence enables just about all other interests and goals.[26] It might, therefore, be argued that the value of life is life itself and not some monetary or other weighting placed upon it by others. On this basis the value of life is inestimable. This 'priceless' view of life has been challenged by Mooney[27] who claims that if life were of infinite value daily living would be impossible as we know it. We take risks daily which imply that the risk of getting knocked down and killed when crossing the road, is for example, a cost not outweighed by the benefits of reaching a shop on the other side of the street. In practice we are prepared to trade-off a higher risk of death than is strictly necessary in order to enjoy some of the good things in life – a personal form of cost-benefit analysis.

Ethically, perhaps the most important principle against which CBA should be assessed is that of justice. The problem with this ideal is the many competing conceptions of justice; justice as rewarding virtue and punishing vice; justice as treating people equally; justice as protecting property and entitlement; justice as ensuring basic needs are satisfied. Economists might argue that distributive justice is achieved best by pursuing economic efficiency but the mainstream ethical theory most closely allied to the economic perspective is Utilitarianism. The principle of utility with its maximisation imperative (of happiness, good or health), provides some ethical justification for the economists' defence of CBA. But the problems of health-status measurement and valuation apply equally to the measurement of utility. A further difficulty arises in the justification of decisions which, although they maximise health overall, result in the deprivation or disadvantage of a minority. The principle introduced by Pareto which states that group welfare is at an optimum when it is impossible to make any one person better off without at the same time making at least one other person worse off has been invoked in an attempt to remedy this dilemma.[28] Economists have engaged in mental gymnastics in order to refine this notion in the form of the 'Hicks-Kaldor test' or the 'potential Pareto-improvement criterion'[29] which creates the theoretical possibility of realizing a Pareto-improvement by the costless redistribution of money. But as with the principle of utility this is actually 'compatible with some persons actually being made worse off, for it requires only a net gain overall'.[30] The problem, too, with the Pareto principle is that to make someone better off without making anyone worse off, merely implies the allocation of resources according to the present pattern to justify the status quo – back to the perpetuation of decibel pressure determined allocations with little or no advantage having been gained from the application of CBA to the problem!

The other application of CBA claimed to be of use is in marginal analysis. An allocation question commonly posed is how much treatment or how much of a particular health-care programme would be worthwhile? Drummond uses the example of day case surgery to illustrate the point.[31] If efficiency is greatest by day case surgery (i.e. equivalent medical effectiveness is obtained at lower cost) but the unit is working to capacity, the treatment of a further ten cases per week may prove more costly because of the extra investment needed to increase resources, than by traditional in-patient management if there is spare capacity in the latter. The primary objection to the consequences of marginal analysis is that to the man at the margin, a ceiling on a particular treatment or place in a health-care programme, is anything but marginal. Harris in his polemic 'The Value of Life'[32] makes it clear that one life is worth one life and that where resources are scarce we should choose between one candidate for care over another in a way which is just and values each citizen equally. The application of marginal analysis implies that individuals seeking assistance at a given point in a treatment programme will be disadvantaged by virtue of an arbitrary ceiling derived from a now discredited cost-benefit analysis. Harris has argued elsewhere that it would be more just (fairer) in such circumstances to toss a coin to determine who should receive the available care.[33]

The CBA approach seems to deny the maxim upon which the Health Service was founded, that of need regardless of ability to pay. The equitable distribution of resources depends on allocation according to need. This principle is clearly illustrated in the system of triage used originally in battle situations as a means of allocating resources to those most in need. Triage has been defined as 'the assignment of the degree of urgency to decide the order treatment of wounds and sickness'.[34] The principle of justice operating in this example permits those with the greatest need (those with the most life threatening pathologies) to be dealt with first, while others, less severely ill, are priority rated and allocated resources accordingly. (The implication if this approach were it to be extended is, of course, that life-saving would take precedence over life-enhancing treatments, but as Harris notes this need not be an absolute imperative because severe pain, discomfort or distress might be worse and require intervention. Life saving as a primary imperative has been discussed above.)

At first glance it might appear that this is CBA operating at the microanalytic (individual patient) level even though Mooney has said that 'it is at a resource planning level that the interest of cost-benefit analysts lies, not individual patient management'.[35] If this is the case, and it seems a morally justifiable system in an emergency, how can it be different from the macroanalytic application of CBA? Superficially it may seem that the only differences are those of scale and immediacy and that moral objections to CBA must therefore be unfounded since it seeks merely to apply the principles tolerated in emergencies to the allocation of resources in all health-care situations. Yet one fundamental difference precludes such a conclusion. In triage no analysis of the benefits (outcome) is undertaken, the allocation of resources is based on assessed need, not on imputed outcome against predicted investment (cost). Thus, the principle of distributive justice according to need prevails over the economic principle of efficiency.

Finally, without resorting to a complete review of his paper, it is worth highlighting some of the criticisms Copp levels at the technique of CBA.[36] He argues that it is unlikely that CBA can take account of the range of costs and benefits it purports to do; that a person's willingness to pay may be a poor measure of the accompanying variation in his welfare (health); that the potential Pareto-improvement ignores the distributional effects of social decisions; that there remains much uncertainty surrounding the rationale of CBA. In outlining three possible rationales of CBA, moralist, rationalist and management science, the first position is closest to the economists' perspective (the efficiency ethic) alluded to in this essay. Copp argues that although CBA is recommended as an aid to the decision maker in reaching an ethical evaluation, 'everyone has a duty to reach ethically acceptable decisions, while not everyone has the responsibility to consult CB analysis'.[37]

There can be little doubt that the choices confronting health-care planners are not to be envied. Recourse to techniques which raise public consciousness and elaborate the facts and considerations to be taken into account in health-care spending can only be applauded – provided such techniques do not seek to deny or distort the moral domain. This essay has explored the moral significance of both CEA and CBA. In comparison the former would appear relatively benign compared to the latter were it not for the fact that both rely entirely on a process of measurement and valuation which purports to be more objective and less value laden than it actually is. Significant problems such as the valuation of human life and the principle of distributive justice have been analysed. The fact remains that the rationale for both CEA and CBA may be spurious. Economic efficiency, whilst applicable in the market place may be an unjustifiable imperative in relation to human lives. Each life is of inestimable value and each life is worth one life. Life saving should take precedence where this does not infringe autonomy since all other goals and interests are subordinate to continued life. No individual can be justifiably disadvantaged other than by chance. These principles are potentially infringed or denied by CBA and to a lesser extent CEA. To paraphrase Copp's statement, decision makers have a duty to reach ethically acceptable solutions in allocating resources for health-care spending but they are not compelled to use CEA or CBA.

Notes

1. G. Mooney, *Economics, Medicine and Health Care* (Brighton: Wheatsheaf Books, 1986) p. 2.
2. R. Maxwell, 'Cutting the Suit According to the Cloth', *The Health Service Journal*, 26 June 1986, ('Centre eight').
3. J. Cumberlege, 'Painful Choices', *Nursing Times* (1 April, 1987) p. 22.
4. Ibid.
5. Mooney, Russell and Weir, *Choices for Health Care* (London: Macmillan, 1980) pp. 40–62.
6. See G. Mooney, *Economics, Medicine and Health Care.*
7. G. Mooney, *Economics, Medicine and Health Care,* p. 14.
8. D. Copp, 'Morality, Reason, and Management Science: The Rationale of Cost-Benefit Analysis', *Social Philosophy and Policy* (Spring 1985) vol. 2, no. 2, p. 130.
9. A. Maynard, Unpublished proceedings of Conference III (1987), M.A. (Philosophy of Health Care). Centre for Philosophy and Health Care, University College, Swansea.
10. Mooney *Economics, Medicine and Health Care.*
11. Mooney, Russell, and Weir, *Choices for Health Care,* p. 49.
12. Drummond, *Principles of Economic Appraisal in Healthe Care* (Oxford: Oxford University Press, 1980) chap. 2.
13. J. A. Muir-Gray, 'Choosing Priorities', *Journal of Medical Ethics* (1979) vol. 5, pp. 73–5.
14. Ibid.
15. J. Cumberlege, 'Painful Choices'.
16. J. Harris, 'Life or Death Debate', *The Health Service Journal,* 26 June 1986, ('Centre eight').
17. Culyer, Lavers and Williams, cited in Mooney, Russell and Weir, *Choices for Health Care,* p. 60.
18. Mooney, *Economics, Medicine and Health Care.*
19. A. Williams, cited in Mooney, Russell and Weir, *Choices for Health Care,* p. 48.
20. Cumberledge, 'Painful Choices'.
21. Mooney, Russell and Weir, *Choices for Health Care* (1980) p. 51.
22. J. A. Muir-Gray, 'Choosing Priorities', p. 73.
23. Mooney, Russell and Weir, *Choices for Health Care,* p. 51.

24. D. Copp, 'Morality, Reason and Management Science', p. 134.
25. C. Fried, 'Distributive Justice', *Social Philosophy and Policy* (1983) vol. 1, no. 1, pp. 46–59.
26. J. Harris, Conference III (1987). M.A. (Philosophy of Health Care). Centre for Philosophy and Health Care, University College, Swansea.
27. G. Mooney, 'Cost-benefit Analysis and Medical Ethics', *Journal of Medical Ethics* (1980) vol. 6, pp. 177–9.
28. J. A. Muir-Gray, 'Choosing Priorities'.
29. D. Copp, 'Morality, Reason and Management Science', p. 131.
30. Ibid.
31. M. F. Drummond, *Principles of Economic Appraisal.*
32. J. Harris, *The Value of Life* (London: Routledge and Kegan Paul, 1985).
33. Ibid.
34. D. K. Brooks, and A. J. Harold, *Modern Emergency Department Practice* (Edward Arnold, 1983).
35. G. H. Mooney, 'Cost-benefit Analysis', p. 178.
36. D. Copp, 'Morality, Reason and Management Science'.
37. Ibid.

9 Experiments on People and Animals

Denise Skiffington

'A man is truly ethical only when he obeys the compunction to help all life he is able to assist, and shrinks from injuring anything that lives . . . life as such is sacred to him. He tears no leaf from a tree, plucks no flower and takes care to crush no insect . . .'[1]

While few of us would hold this rather extreme view on 'reverence for life' that formed an essential part of the philosophy of Albert Schweitzer, most would agree that there is something 'special' about living things that demands a respect not afforded inanimate objects, and that there is something particularly special about human life that sets it apart again from other living entities. But what is it that places human life on such a lofty pedestal? Are there any rational grounds for making this assumption which, after all, forms one of the most basic premises around which human society operates? An appreciation of the moral status of life, human and non-human, is, I believe, fundamental to the question under consideration, for it is only then that one can approach individual issues such as the ethics of experimentation on any logical basis.

That much controversy still surrounds when 'life' actually begins and ends does not preclude ascribing moral status to it. Indeed, an understanding of the moral significance of 'life' is a crucial element in attempts to unravel this very dilemma. Consideration of this issue, though of profound importance, will not be given coverage in this essay. The western traditional view of the importance of 'being human' is seen by many to be a blend of Greek, Jewish and Christian influences, with all three agreeing that humans occupy a special place in creation. Reasons offered by Judaeo-Christianity are of course based in religious beliefs. Man was made in the image of God and thus must be shown great deference and respect. Man, as opposed to any other living being, was given a soul, the presence of which renders his body a 'temple of the Holy Spirit' and the nature of which is immortal.

Further, we must respect human life simply because God respects it. Such views are entirely dependent on faith and thus neither scientifically verifiable nor founded in rationality. The value of life becomes grounded in the value God places on it and is thus dependent on its relationship with Him rather than on something inherent in itself. Does this therefore mean that if one does not believe in God one need not place a value on life, because after all, its value only derives from its relationship with him?

Edward Shils regards it as self-evident that life is sacred. Hans Jonas concurs by writing: '[life], is believed to be sacred not because it is a manifestation of a transcendent creator, but because it is life. The idea of sacredness is generated by the primordial experience of being alive, of experiencing the elemental fear of existence . . .'[2] Thus for Shils all life, not only human, has a 'sanctity' deserving of respect. While religious contribution to the concept of 'sanctity of human life' is very powerful and duly noted, it does seem to offer, at best, inadequate and implausible grounds for affording human life the elevated position it enjoys in the hierarchy of the animal world, and for explaining the respect for life usually demonstrated by other members of the species.

What is needed is a rational and logically consistent approach to 'moral consideration', such that we may develop a closer understanding of the scope of moral respect and of the beings, human and otherwise, that are deserving of our moral attention. Thomas Aquinas'[3] view was that: 'Other creatures are for the sake of the intellectual creatures . . . and further . . . that hence it is not wrong for man to make use of them (dumb animals) either by killing or in any other way . . .' Kant[4] held the view that 'humanity in virtue of its rational nature is an end in itself' and that . . . 'animals are there merely as a means to an end and that end is man . . .'. Thus many centuries after Aristotle suggested it, Kant was concurring that man's uniqueness lay in his rationality. An immediate problem exists with choosing 'rationality' as the property which sets human life apart. How does one treat those who are not rational – the babes, the mental retards and the comatose? Are they only afforded the same status as 'non-humans', or is one to presume that the extent to which such proponents consider human life to be unique is determined rather by the norm for the species rather than individual performances?

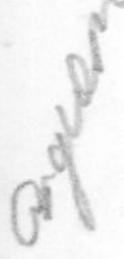

Nor is it evident that all animals lack the capacity to manifest at least some of the mental powers hitherto attributed only to man. There is a growing literature in comparative psychology that indicates that at least some animals are capable of forms of intentionality, reasoning and language, albeit primitive. Interestingly both Kant and Aquinas agree that cruelty to animals is wrong, but only because it may lead to similar cruelty to humans.

Warnock dismisses the criterion of rationality as intolerably narrow, and offers, 'that the condition of being a proper beneficiary of moral action, is the capacity of suffering the ills of the predicament . . .'.[5] Jeremy Bentham also pointed to the capacity for suffering as the vital characteristic that gives a being the right to moral consideration, and Peter Singer with his high profile anti-vivisectionist attitude states that 'if a being is not capable of suffering or of experiencing enjoyment or happiness, there is nothing to be taken into account.'[6]

Such convictions are laudable and on the surface seem to offer a reasonable criterion for moral consideration. After all, inflicting pain is a damnable act, no matter against whom it is perpetrated. Certainly the capacity to suffer is a good reason for showing moral concern towards a being, but is it a necessary prerequisite? Before going any further I feel that there is an important distinction which must be appreciated and that is between an entity having 'moral worth' and being a 'moral agent'. As Caplan points out, what may be sufficient in terms of properties that concern moral worth or standing are hardly sufficient in terms of properties that confer moral agency and moral responsibility.[7] What we are concerned with at the moment is trying to define these 'moral objects' and to determine the characteristics (if possible) which make such beings 'morally considerable'. Caplan's own opinion is that 'purposiveness' (having basic drives, desires and intentions) is the property that suffices to confer moral worth. To return to the suggestion that the capacity to suffer/enjoy (or sentience) confers moral worth on creatures and more specifically to Singer's viewpoint. He believes that if a being is not capable of sentience 'there is nothing to be taken into account', and that the capacity for sentience is a 'prerequisite for having interests at all'.

Again I have difficulty interpreting 'capacity'. If he means the actual ability of each individual to suffer/enjoy, then a section of humanity, albeit very small, is 'not worth taking into account' and thus expendable. I refer to those human beings damaged neurologically in such a way as to be totally unresponsive. Is

Singer saying that they 'have no interests' or are we once again floundering in the realms of 'potential capacity' and norm for the species?

From a biological point of view, sentience appears to be an adaptive characteristic of living things providing them with a better capacity to anticipate and avoid life-threatening situations. As Goodpaster suggests, this at least allows for the possibility that 'the capacity to suffer and enjoy are ancillary to something more important, rather than tickets to considerability in their own right'.[8] Or in the words of a perceptive observer . . . 'the pleasure signal is only an evolutionary derived indicator, not the goal itself'.

So far I have looked at various theories for placing human life on an elevated plateau, as well as examining some of the criteria deemed sufficient for conferring moral worth on an entity. While I agree that rationality, sentience, intelligence and purpose are all good reasons for so doing, I do not see them as essential prerequisites. I, like Goodpaster, believe that the presence of 'life' alone is sufficient, though hasten to add that I am aware of the many dissenters and of the sort of objections they tender. Before proceeding to the thorny particulars of experimentation, I will briefly counter some of the more common objections to the 'life principle'.

Suggesting that moral considerability is synonomous and coexistent with life, is interpreted by some as meaning that feeling, thinking humans are thus of no more moral consequence than a cabbage or mouse. These people miss the crucial difference I referred to earlier; that between moral objects and moral agents. I am not suggesting that mice and dogs, because they should be afforded moral consideration, can in any way be expected to display moral responsibility towards others. This is one of the things that does set man apart – because of his intellectual, rational but more importantly, his moral attributes, man is not only deserving of moral consideration, but must accept moral responsibility for his own actions, (something which other living beings cannot) and must be prepared to acknowledge and respect the 'rights' of other living beings.

If we lived in an ideal world, this would mean allowing all living things to pursue their aims unobstructed and live out their lives without risk of interference from man. But we do not live in Utopia, and so if man is to survive and conquer disease in this world of limited resources and conflicting purposes (a 'speciesist' attitude, according to Singer), he must eat, though not necessarily meat and he must continue to seek ways to fulfil this end. That some animals may have to suffer on the way seems almost inevitable, but I will return to this later. I am not suggesting for a moment that this 'right to life' is an absolute; but if we are to interfere with and abrogate what is a prima facie right to live and be left alone, we must provide compelling reasons for so doing.

Yet others may hold that since one cannot offer a precise definition of 'life' it cannot be used as a criterion for considerability. As I stated earlier, while the definition of life and its boundaries is fraught with difficulties it does not preclude ascribing it moral status. As Goodpaster says, 'surely rationality, potential rationality, sentience and the possession of interests fare no better'.

And so to experimentation. Having decided that all living things deserve moral consideration and respect, how does this relate to experimentation, and to the differences, if any, between the use of humans and non-humans in such experiments? I will be concerned largely with the area of bio-medical research but wish to touch briefly on two other areas initially. The use of animals in research related to cosmetics is a heinous activity and one to be deplored. Inflicting pain on any creature simply to satisfy the vanity of humans is indefensible. Similarly the poor conditions under which many farm animals are bred in order to provide their owners with large profits and the public with the sort of produce they desire is again inexcusable and I believe morally corrupt. But when it comes to the area of bio-medical research, the issue becomes clouded.

The aims of such research are ostensibly altruistic – the improvement of health and the saving of lives (human lives of course); with the assumption that the acquisition of such knowledge will always lead to improved care. There are many who question if there is any substantial evidence to prove this. Indeed, Illitch believes that 'doctors have affected epidemics (in the past century) . . . no more profoundly than did priests in earlier times', and further, that the approach to research is responsible for 'the present endemic health denial'.[9]

While the whole question of the moral legitimacy of such experimentation is a topic in itself, it obviously needs to be addressed to some extent in this work. Indeed, if there can be no moral justification for research then the nature of the subjects becomes an irrelevance. There can be no denying that fighting disease and premature death are fine goals – but at what cost? No longer is the 'advancement' of the human condition relegated to the sometime fortuitous efforts of a few highly motivated humanitarian scientists – it has become a societal demand. The expectation of the public is that research will continue to prove and solve the still unanswered questions while generally aiming to promote and improve the human lot wherever possible. As The Black Report states, 'Achieving a high standard of health among it's people represents one of the highest of society's aspirations.'[10] In order to fulfil this onerous responsibility, there is an obvious need for research. That such research must involve man as experimental subject would seem to be an essential part of the process if the new drug/technique is to be adequately assessed in the population who will benefit from it.

But can we justify using animals as experimental subjects, when they have nothing at all to gain and quite a lot to lose? The dilemma becomes one of a conflict of interests between two groups of 'morally considerable' entities – man's desire and right to the best standard of health possible and the animal's desire and right to be left alone and alive. If we are to pursue medical research, and I believe it is morally justifiable and a moral responsibility, then unless we are prepared to use large numbers of humans in the various and some potentially dangerous stages of its pursuit, there seems little alternative but to use animals. Attempts are being made to develop alternatives to the use of live subjects, but this is at an early stage and not a feasible proposition at the moment, though one that holds promise for the future and one that should be pursued earnestly. Singer might say that it is a 'speciesist' attitude which holds that animals should be sacrificed in the interests of human welfare and to a certain degree this is so. We are making the decision that in order of rank of considerability, human interests outweigh those of animals. This ranking of priorities appears to be an inevitable part of moral existence.

So to the question of which animals to use. There are some restrictions imposed by the nature of the research itself, but as a general rule it would seem appropriate to use animals from the lowest phylogenetic scale when possible. This does not mean in any way that these creatures, however simple in construction, should not be afforded the respect due to all living things. Indeed, it could be said that we have a special responsibility towards such creatures because they are unable to protect themselves and are so utterly dependent on humans for alleviating the suffering they encounter. We are morally obliged to minimise the numbers of animals used, avoid duplication and to keep pain and suffering at an absolute minimum. For 'the evil of pain is, in itself, unaffected by the other characteristics of the being that feels that pain; the value of life is affected by these other characteristics'. These other characteristics Singer was referring to include self-awareness, intelligence and the capacity for meaningful relationships with others. Such features become crucial when we have to consider the relative value to place on human versus animal life, but are quite irrelevant to the question of pain.

Having decided that it is morally justifiable to use animals in research, an enormous responsibility is implicit. Caplan[11] believes, and I am in agreement, that 'There must be strict guidelines within which the researcher must act, but if we, the public, demand the benefits seen to be gained from such work, then we must also accept the responsibility for ensuring that it is carried out with due regard to the animal's sensibilities.' For it is 'only out of ignorance and expediency that we put members of the animal kingdom to our purpose rather than theirs'.

The use of human experimental subjects raises a potentially new set of considerations and ethical problems. Not only are humans morally considerable, (and thus entitled to similar considerations afforded their non-human counterparts), but they are moral agents with moral standing, rights and responsibilities, which place them in a uniquely vulnerable position. The 'common good', or societal interest may become pitted against the interests of the individual, and in order for exploitation not to occur one must be aware of the potentialities. I have suggested that research is ethically justifiable and perhaps even morally obligatory, but that does not mean carte blanche for the experimenters. If society demands continual progress then there seems no alternative but to use human subjects in at least some stages of the tests – but society must be prepared to count the inevitable cost of this trade-off between conflicting interests; those of the perceived benefit to society as a whole, and to the integrity and autonomy of the individual.

Freedom of choice is a highly prized endowment. Can we ensure that those who agree to take part in experimentation have done so entirely freely and without coercion? Should we as individuals feel obligated to make such sacrifices in the interest of future society because we feel indebted to those who have made such gestures in the past? R. M. Hare refers to this as 'moral inducement'. Moreover, do we have a duty to society in this regard? Having a right to the ultimate benefits of medical research does not of itself imply obligations on the right holder, and so participating should be free of all social pressure and opted for 'freely'. But as Jonas states, the mere issuing of an appeal and calling for volunteers inevitably generates moral and social pressures and amount to a sort of conscripting, even with the most meticulous attention to the principles of freedom of choice and consent.[12] I can see no way round this. There will always be individuals who feel 'obliged' to make a contribution to society in the absence of any sort of pressure – 'it's the least I can do' attitude. We are all victims of social conditioning and even the donation of money to a charity, while being totally up to the individual and thus 'free', is all bound up with how we perceive our obligations and duties to others. But can you call it coercion?

Gerald Dworkin argues that an individual is acting freely, i.e. is not coerced, if he does not mind doing 'that action for that reason'.[13] So when I give money to a charity I am acting freely; but I am not acting freely when I give money to kidnappers if I object to so doing in order to secure the release of my son. But there is an obvious flaw in this stance. All arguments could be reinterpreted in such a way that the person always does what he wants to do and is therefore never coerced. Thus when I give money to the kidnappers I am still doing what I want to do, i.e. saving my son's life; and when the prisoner agrees to take part in research he is doing what he wants to do, i.e. securing his early release or contributing to his own welfare by way of money received.

But even if one does accept this redescription and reinterpretation, there is another sense in which the prisoner has not made a free choice, and that is according to Joel Feinberg's[14] idea of 'dispositional liberty'. According to this, a person is free only if he can do considerably more than he wants to do. So in order to be making a free choice in this sense, the prisoner must have been offered alternatives and thus been able to choose otherwise. Clearly the use of prisoners in research is open to more potential abuse simply because they are a 'captive audience', and thus the threats versus offers versus free choice issue is more critical.

My first impression is that no prisoner should be used in experimentation because it is impossible to gauge the amount of coercion and threat involved, be it real, or perceived. But while I recognise that the prisoner is in a peculiarly vulnerable position and does require perhaps even greater protection than the public at large, there are other aspects to be addressed. Presume for the moment that the prisoner has been able to give 'free' consent; there is now an additional moral question as to whether he or she should be allowed to gain benefits by participating. The answer to this will depend largely on one's concept of punishment. For the retributive theory it might be argued that a certain punishment is mandatory and that any alteration to this would be inappropriate.

The issue then becomes one of limits of punishment. Is it only denial of liberty or other deprivations as well – money, self-respect and self-esteem, all of which he could gain as a result of taking part in research. So should we deny the prisoner the possibility or opportunity of elevating his self-worth and thus contributing to his own rehabilitation? Clearly these are issues more concerned with justice and the morality of punishment, and while I think them worthy of note, they do not alter my belief that because of the high risk of exploitation, prisoners should not be used as research subjects.

The issue of consent just raised is one of the most controversial and one that is obviously peculiar to the use of human subjects. Legal requirement is for a free and fully informed consent, emphasised in the Declaration of Helsinki and which on the surface seems to offer a powerful safeguard for the individual's rights. But determining what constitutes such a consent continues to pose problems for experimenter and ethicist alike. In some ways, it seems like a mythical and unattainable ideal, while in its strictest terms, it is an impossibility. If, indeed, the consent was 'fully informed', i.e. the subject was aware of all the risks/benefits, there would be no need to proceed with the research, since to determine these very features is the rationale for much experimentation. But unless we wish research to cease because we consider this goal unattainable, we must find some middle ground.

The overriding moral concern behind the issue of consent must be respect for the subject's autonomy and personal integrity; but while providing the ethical guidelines within which the researcher must operate, this offers no solution to the practical difficulties encountered. How informed and informable should the subject be? Let me concentrate for the moment on non-therapeutic research on adults who have as far as is feasible, 'freely' consented to participate. If we are to 'fully inform' these people of the risks/benefits of the procedure, then clearly those best suited and least likely to be exploited would be intelligent, motivated people, preferably with a scientific background. But this would drastically reduce the number of available subjects and thus prove an impediment to scientific pursuit. So the catchment area must be widened but with obvious limitations. Those involved should be intellectually able to grasp the nature of the work, thus excluding any with intellectual handicap who could, of course, be open to abuse.

But much investigation has shown that despite detailed information being given to subjects, their level of comprehension and retention is poor. Inglefinger[15] says that the 'trouble with informed consent is that it is not educated consent'. He goes on to say that extensive detail enhances the subject's confusion and quotes Epstein and Lasagna who showed that comprehension of medical information given to untutored subjects, is inversely correlated with the elaborateness of the material presented. Justice Kirby of the Australian Law Reform Commission found in one group of cancer patients, that only 60 per cent understood the purpose and nature of a procedure to which they had agreed, while only 40 per cent had read the consent form carefully.[16] There is still a powerful belief that 'doctor knows best', such that patients will offer themselves up with the presumption that the doctor/researcher will always have their best interests at heart.

Bernard Barber suggests that the struggle for scientific priority and recognition, exerts pressure on ethical consideration and that his data shows 'the social structure of competition and reward is one of the sources of permissive experimentation with human subjects'.[17] He concludes his article by stating that since professional power is based largely on knowledge not yet available to the public, it must in some degree be self-regulated; but that since this power is of such public consequence, it must also be subject to significant public control. The establishment of ethics committees has been some attempt to address this responsibility, but the constitution of such groups has been frequently open to question. They usually consist of an abundance of scientific/medical personnel, coupled with what often seems like the token member of the clergy and/or legal profession. If such bodies are to perform their task effectively and be morally accountable, there must first be a balance between the scientific members and those who are objectively representing the interests of the potential subjects.

Returning to animal experimentation momentarily, the passing of the Animal (Scientific Procedures) Act 1986 now appears to afford animals far more protection than did the 1876 Act. A dual licensing system has come into practice whereby a compulsory personal licence of competence as well as a project licence is required by the senior member of each research team. The species and number of animals is also to be specified. The Act does not ban specific experiments (a fact which has brooked some criticism), but rather attempts to exert some control on all aspects of research. As such, it is a welcome addition to the armamentarium against unethical practices.

Before bringing this essay to a close, I will make brief reference to two important issues. Randomised clinical trials (RCT) pose real ethical dilemmas. How ethical is it to give one group of patients (who are particularly vulnerable simply because of illness) a potentially dangerous treatment for example, while possibly denying another group a beneficial one? On the other hand, how will one ever determine what is the best treatment if such trials are not performed, and moreover, is there a moral duty to continue with them? Phillips and Dawson believe that the essential safeguard for the patient in such cases, is again, informed consent.[18] That the patient must freely agree to the work is not disputed (though Brewin from The Institute of Radiotherapeutics states that since randomised treatment is not research, but an attempt to find the best treatment for the patient, consent can be dispensed with), but again the thorny question arises of how informed they should be.

Should they, for example, be told that their therapy is being determined by some randomising procedure rather than their own doctor's personal judgement? Some scientists argue that such information could affect the outcome of the work while others agree that it is essential information which should be imparted. But as Fried points out, a physician has a duty to inform his patient if his broken leg is not healing and that there was another method of treatment available in a nearby city which was more likely to result in cure.[19] Surely this doctrine is equally applicable to a participant in an RCT whose treatment is proving less successful than an alternative.

On the subject of the use of children in research I will be brief, though the topic is vast and deserving of singular consideration. The report from the working committee of the Institute of Medical Ethics released recently, offers clear guidelines.[20] Again the area of consent poses difficulties. Will parents and guardians always have the best interests of their children at heart? Consider the Jehovah

Witness parents who refuse a blood transfusion for their child – in this instance the decision is taken out of their hands. But if we then say that parents across the board cannot be trusted to act in the interests of their offspring, do we not undermine the importance of parents? The recommendation by the working party that parents should only be considered trustees of a child's interests rather than having rights over them is welcome. It is perhaps in the area of child research, both therapeutic and non-therapeutic, that well constituted and enthusiastic ethics committees are most vital.

Thus the use of both human and non-human in research is beset with many dilemmas; some shared between the two groups and others peculiar to only one. I have stated that all living creatures are morally considerable for that reason alone and must be afforded respect commensurate with this property. Humans, by virtue of their status as moral agents who are free to make choices and who have moral responsibilities towards themselves and others, invite a whole new set of problems related to consent, freedom of choice and personal autonomy. Pitted against all of which are the interests and advancement of society. Caplan states that animal experimentation 'is always morally tragic. No matter what goods are promoted by the process, some creatures who are unable to alter their circumstances, will have their basic rights to life and fulfilment infringed'.[21] Hans Jonas offers a final caveat: 'Let us not forget that progress is an optional goal, not an unconditional commitment, and that its tempo, compulsive as it may become, has nothing sacred about it.'[22]

Notes

1. O. Temkin, W. Frankena and S. Kadish *Respect for Life in Medicine, Philosophy and the Law* (Johns Hopkins University Press, 1977) p. 56.
2. Ibid., pp. 30–1.
3. See J. Rachels, *The End of Life-Euthanasia and Morality* (Oxford: Oxford University Press, 1977) pp. 13–14.
4, See Rachels, ibid., p. 13
5. G. J. Warnock, *The Object of Morality* (New York: Methuen, 1971).
6. P. Singer, *Animal Liberation* (New York: Avon Books, 1977).
7. A. Caplan, *Beastly Conduct – Ethical Issues in Animal Experimentation* (New York: Academy of Science, 1983) pp. 159–69.
8. K. Goodpaster, 'On Being Morally Considerable', *Journal of Philosophy* (1975) pp. 308–24.

9. P. Illitch, *Medical Nemesis* (Calder & Boyars, 1975).
10. P. Townsend and W. Davidson, *Inequalities in Health. The Black Report* (Harmondsworth: Penguin, 1982).
11. Ibid.
12. H. Jonas, 'Philosophical Fluctuations on Experimenting with Human Subjects', in P. Freund, *Experimentation with Human Subjects* (American Academy of Arts and Sciences, 1970).
13. G. Dworkin, 'Acting Freely', *Novs* vol. 4, pp. 367–83.
14. J. Feinberg, *Social Philosophy* (Englewood Cliffs: Prentice Hall, 1973).
15. F. Inglefinger, 'Informed (but Uneducated) Consent', *New England Journal of Medicine* (1987).
16. *Respect for Life in Medicine Philosophy and the Law* (Johns Hopkins University Press, 1977).
17. B. Barber, 'The Ethics of Experimentation with Human Subjects', *Scientific American*, vol. 234, no. 2, pp. 25–31.
18. M. Phillips and J. Dawson, *Doctors' Dilemmas, Medical Ethics and Contemporary Science* (Brighton: Harvester Press, 1985).
19. C. Fried, *Medical Experimentation Personal Intergrity and Social Policy* (American Elsevier Pub., 1974).
20. 'Medical Research with Children. Ethics Law and Practice', *IME Bulletin* (May 1986) pp. 8–9.
21. Ibid.
22. H. Jonas, ibid.

10 The Development of Drugs

Paul Goulden

The dictionary definition of drug is 'A medical substance used alone or as an ingredient'. Although in common usage 'drug' tends to be associated with illegal stimulants, I will use it here to mean any substance administered with a view to producing physiological change (excluding the basic metabolic requirements of food, water and oxygen). The physiological change may be therapeutic in itself or merely facilitate a therapeutic procedure (e.g. anaesthesia), it may be preventative (e.g. immunisation), or palliative. The effect may be either direct on the target individual or by moderating the effect of some parasitic organism (e.g. anti-microbials). Thus the field of what can be called a drug is vast, from Acyclovir to Zovirax, from the simplest natural compound to the most complex product of genetic engineering or organic chemistry.

I do not intend to discuss the dominant role of drugs in modern medical practice. Although often founded on unproved theories, alternative therapies such as acupuncture and manipulation have a role, but drugs will occupy centre stage for a long time yet. On the basis that there is still a need for new drugs and better ways of using the ones we have, I wish to consider the ethical aspects of the drug development process. The development of a drug falls, as I see it, into four distinct parts, and in each case the ethical position is far from being as clear cut as those of us who prescribe drugs everyday, or reach for an aspirin when we have a headache, might wish.

The four stages are the initial test tube work, animal experiments, tests on human volunteers or non-ill subjects and clinical trials in patients. Each stage presents its own problems, and I intend to look at each in turn.

The initial, test tube, stage of drug development seems ethically very straightforward at first. We have a happy image of the school chemistry laboratory or Alexander Fleming with his mouldy petri dish and imagine modern drug research is like that. Of course it is not. It is a sophisticated multi-million pound process in which drugs are tailored to have molecular shapes to fit known receptors and scores of chemicals are synthesised to find one with the desired properties. The system consumes vast amounts of finance and skilled manpower. 'Fine, more power to their elbow!' After all they are working to conquer disease. Or are they?

On a global scale the vast majority of disease is caused by nutritional and environmental factors. The discovery of new drugs is an irrelevance to these; to give anti-bacterial therapy to someone with a contaminated water supply seems a strange approach. Even if we confine our discussion to the economically developed world where malnutrition, polluted water and overcrowding play a much smaller role in the disease process (although inexcusably they are not completely unknown), there is much in the environment, eating patterns and life style, such as smoking, which could be changed with benefit to health.

However, attention to these matters will not abolish disease, at least not in the short term, and while some measures are of proven benefit, in other cases it is not clear exactly what should be done. How much more exercise, fibre or meditation? How much less atmospheric lead, saturated fat or gamma radiation? Therefore, there is and will be a role for drugs in the health process. An ethical difficulty is in deciding what these drugs should be.

Modern drugs (post-Second World War) have been researched and developed almost entirely by multi-national corporations based in Europe and the USA. The role of publicly funded bodies such as universities and the Medical Research Council seems to be more in basic science or in evaluating the products of drug houses. It may be that the resources available to any single non-commercial research group are simply not on the same scale as those available to a drug company, or attitudes may be different. Suffice it to say that non-commercial sources are not delivering the goods. That said, why are the drug companies financing drug development?

The only answer is to produce a marketable product and from its sales not only recoup their cost, but produce a profit for their shareholders. It would be odd if this were not so, as this is the purpose of corporate endeavour in a capitalist society. If you can relieve suffering or cure cancer, great, but that by itself is not the name of the game. This puts an immediate limitation on lines of development it is worth pursuing. What is required is either a very common condition, so that a lot of drugs can be sold (and if it is not a permanent cure, even better), or one which is so serious and emotive that a high price will be paid for treatment.

An example of the former approach is drugs for the treatment of hypertension. There is no agreement over the level of hypertension which should be treated to avoid complications. However, everybody has a blood pressure and in some it is higher than others, hence hypertension seems like a winner. In addition, no drug has been produced which in a single dose or short course, reduces blood pressure and keeps it down. Therapy must be lifelong. In addition, hypertension is often asymptomatic, so there is not the troublesome problem of patients stopping treatment because they feel better. Given this, is it any surprise that there are over seventy formulations in the UK market which list treatment of hypertension as one of their indications (excluding variable dose and route versions of the same product)?

Contrast this with, say, amoebiasis, not only uncommon in the UK, but curable. Less than half a dozen preparations are available, and some of these of limited value. Equally, nobody seems very interested in using interferon to treat the common cold!

This said, does this approach pose any ethical problem? Do drug houses have any responsibility to society or should they just respond to commercial pressures? It could be argued that the money they spend on research is not their own, but has been taken from the consumer by price mark-ups on individual drugs. There may be a difference of over one hundred per cent in the cost of a drug from a company which only manufactures established lines and one which runs a research and development programme. Is this extra money more appropriately spent on developing treatments for conditions where existing therapy is poor or non-existent or in developing 'next-generation' antibiotics, antihypertensives and tranquillisers when the existing products have barely been evaluated?

In addition to the financial responsibilities of the drug house, there are manpower implications. In any society there must be a limit to the number of scientists who can be educated, and the number of truly original thinkers is small indeed. If drug companies are able to seduce them by paying 'top-dollars' and then put them to work playing molecular roulette to produce 'me too' drugs, are they making the most appropriate use of a scarce resource? However, having produced a number of promising looking compounds the ethical problems really start as we move on to stage two of the development procedure, invariably animal tests.

Both government legislation and public sentiment in western countries (which are all we are really talking about, so far as serious drug research is concerned), demand animal testing before a drug is used in humans. Apart from the relevance and value of some of the tests, there is a strong philosophical case against using animals as experimental subjects at all, and I would like to digress for a few moments to consider this.

The use of animals for whatever humans wish has a long and not very honourable history in western society. Indeed, in the Holy Bible man is given 'dominion over the fish of the sea, and the fowl of the air and over every living thing that liveth upon the earth'. By the time of Jesus the situation had not changed, for despite mentioning that 'God feedeth the fowls of the air', a herd of swine is seen as a conventional repository for dispossessed devils. (It must be said that eastern religions, particularly those which preach reincarnation often have a very different attitude to animals.)

Apart from the Bible, and long custom and practice, what is the basis of our use of animals, either for experimentation or food, and does it amount to exploitation? This is a question which increasingly troubles the general public although it is by no means new as a subject of philosophical thought. Descartes and Jeremy Bentham both pronounced on the subject (although their views were almost totally opposed).

In this age of equality and 'ISMISM', different treatment should be based on different characteristics, and significantly different ones at that. If it is not acceptable to differentiate on the basis of anatomical differences (sexism) or skin colour (racism), what is such a big deal about being a human which can avoid the charge of 'speciesism'?

Given that animals, at least the higher ones, have a nervous system and brain similar to a human's, albeit with a less developed neocortex, it is not surprising that it is hard to name an ability of importance which is not either found in animals as well as man or is absent in a sufficiently high number of humans to remove its value as a discriminator. In particular it is difficult to avoid removing infants, the elderly and the mentally handicapped to a sort of 'honorary human' status, granted because they have two arms, two legs and a smooth(ish) skin, but are otherwise philosophically no different from animals.

Frey believes that language is the key difference. He apparently believes that, if I cannot say to myself 'I have a pain', I don't have one, whatever I may feel and whatever other evidence, such as autonomic arousal there may be. This is as improbable as Descartes emphasis on reason, 'Cogito ergo sum', and for much the same reason. The concept of language or even reason as the discriminating factor rules out millions for whom they are only a potential, a memory or not even a possibility (because of mental handicap) from consideration as members of the elite human group. Frey dismisses this mass of people as marginal cases, not worthy of further consideration, but the strength of a theory rests on how well it works for marginal cases. Once there is a margin there is the possibility of the border moving and it seems odd that the very groups we wish to protect from exploitation can be classified as only marginally different from animals we can exploit willy-nilly.

For some people Bentham correctly identified the question as 'not can they reason, nor can they talk, but can they suffer?' Most people however fall back on an apologetically 'speciesist', RSPCA sort of stance, and say we accept exploitation of animals, defining animals on a crude 'four legged and hairy' basis, but would like suffering to be kept to a minimum. Animal experiments therefore, we will have.

Some animal experimentation takes place to elucidate basic physiological or psychological principles. I will not consider this further but will concentrate on procedures associated with developing a new drug. Animal tests in this situation fall into two groups, 'does it work?' and 'is it toxic?' The 'does it work group' in which the new 'designer molecule' is given to animals to see if it has the desired effect, produces immediate problems.

If the effect is one which can be produced in the normal individual and has a clearly defined end point, it is clear what is needed. Straightforward experiments can take place, under anaesthesia if appropriate. Either a muscle relaxant produces paralysis, or a diuretic a diuresis, or it does not. However, supposing the change can only take place in abnormal specimens, for example the healing of ulcers. The animal needs to be manipulated to produce a condition similar to that the drug is aimed at in humans. This may involve suffering, and may not even provide a particularly appropriate model. For instance, primates can be given duodenal ulcers by repeated exposure to electric shocks. It is hard to imagine that this does not cause suffering, and it does not work if performed under anaesthesia. Similarly, diabetic dogs are not commonly available, and the recovery from pancreatectomy is not likely to be any more pleasant for a dog than it is for a man.

Because of the difficulties in providing adequate animal models for many of the conditions the drug companies are interested in, because of their sales potential, such as mild hypertension, depression and rheumatoid arthritis, this type of animal study cannot always be undertaken. The law requires that toxicity tests be performed, although their relevance to the human situation is not always obvious.

Testing for acute cellular toxicity can be carried out on tissue culture material. If the compound disrupts cell structure there is not much point in pursuing it further. This approach does not seem to present many ethical problems apart from the minor one of the right of ownership of human derived cell lines. The greater part of drug toxicity testing must be carried out on whole animals, and it is here again that moral problems arise. Even if exploitation of animals is to be allowed, how is suffering to be minimised?

A popular test, at least with drug licensing authorities, is the so called LD 50 test, in which the dose of drug required to kill half of a group of test animals is determined. This may then be compared with therapeutic doses to provide an index of safety. This approach may have some validity in testing a drug such as digitalis where the toxic dose is of the same order of magnitude as the therapeutic dose and death is fairly quick due to cardiac standstill.

Supposing, however, that this is not the case, and we are testing, say, an antibiotic? The chances are that this would not produce death at a dose anything like the effective dose, and death would probably not be from sudden cardiac arrest, but might be from, say, aplastic anaemia. What in these circumstances would be the value of poisoning a group of animals, all of whom might become very ill before half of them died. It would not be possible to use anaesthetics or analgesics lest these confuse the results. Furthermore, there is more to toxicity than sudden death, so a group of animals must be sacrificed for post-mortem examination for tumours, ulcers and so on.

The relevance of drug testing in animals is further thrown into question by species specificity. This can lead to false assurance or erroneous doubts. Thalidomide never caused phocomelia in animals in which it was tested prior to marketing. Guinea pigs die when given penicillin and laboratory animals are so inbred that some have a high spontaneous incidence of abnormalities. Often human studies are commenced before animal work is complete. The patent life of a drug is short, so it must be tempting to press on once it is clear that your animals are not going to keel over after the first few doses, rather than watch them eat it without harm for years.

There is no law to prevent anything being administered to a consenting adult volunteer and here again we run into problems of paternalism, exploitation and respect for autonomy. Initial drug testing in humans is undertaken in volunteers. However, their method of selection, and the fact that they generally receive a payment sometimes called expenses, calls into question the genuinely free nature of their participation.

Subjects are generally recruited from students and laboratory staff. It may well be that some participate against their better judgement in order to please their superiors and appear to be pulling their weight. Indeed students are so eager to please that it is perfectly possible to disguise drug trials as class practicals. It is very difficult for a student with little training in medicine or pharmacology to seriously question a senior researcher about a study.

The payment of 'expenses' puts further pressure on students as the amount usually significantly enhances their income. This could lead to abuse, such as taking part in trials they are not happy with, or when they are not well, or even taking part in two trials simultaneously.

A further problem is the question of liability if anything serious befalls the subject who is legally neither a patient nor an employee. Volunteer drug tests often take place at one remove from the developing company, either in university departments or commercial test houses, so the legal situation is complex.

Volunteer studies are necessarily limited both in length and result. They tend to look for acute symptoms, changes in the blood picture and so on. Students are a relatively transient population, so long-term follow up is difficult. Not many would submit to tests as invasive as, say, liver biopsy, and obviously autopsy material is not (usually) available. Volunteer studies are very poor predictors of longer term problems.

Students and similar young people may be poor models for the group of patients the drug is intended for. The impaired metabolism of old age may allow the drug to accumulate in a way not seen in the young. The possibility of the aggravation of pre-existing disease, or interaction with other medications cannot be assessed. The testing of drugs for their effects on human pregnancy is a particularly difficult area. Therefore it may not be possible to be completely truthful about all the effects of a drug before applying for a clinical trial certificate (necessary in this country), and going on to trials in real patients, suffering from the problem the drug is designed for.

Under the terms of the Helsinki declaration, which itself is based on the Nuremberg code, consent to participate in a trial should be freely given and informed. However, patients are generally in a dependent position to their physician and are quite likely to participate just to please, without fully appreciating that the choice is theirs.

It is easy to be paternalistic over the question of informed consent and assume the patient will not understand explanation of the aims, objects, methods and risk of the study. Answers to some of their questions may not even be possible. There is particular pressure to participate if the new drug is held out as an advance. ('It must be, otherwise they wouldn't be testing. Would they?')

At particular risk of coercive consent are patients with conditions such as depression, where existing treatment is not completely successful and dependence on the physician can be very high. It is doubtful if truly informed consent can ever be obtained in these circumstances. Similarly difficult is the validity of proxy consent for children and mental incompetents. Clearly it is not possible to avoid testing drugs on these groups if conditions specific to them are to be treated, but the problems are considerable.

Drug trials should be scrutinised by an independent ethical committee. There has been a tendency for these to adopt a paternalistic view and support the rights of the man pushing forward the frontiers of science over those of the patient. A sort of utilitarian argument may be used to support this 'What if the rights of a few are impaired a little bit if this treatment will benefit millions?'

The favoured type of drug trial is double blind, in which neither the doctor nor the patient know what drug is being used, the code being held by a third party and allocated at random. This produces two problems. First if the drug is an improvement on its predecessors, is it not an affront to the autonomy of the individual to let a computer decide if he should have it. Secondly, it is common practice not to ask patients to participate in the trial until after randomisation. This is wrong, as the randomisation is actually part of the trial procedure.

In conclusion, it can be seen that the development and testing of drugs is an ethical minefield in which the commercial interests of companies, the rights of animals and the autonomous rights of individuals must all be considered. These may be in conflict. For instance people may want more animal tests before taking the drug themselves, animal rightists may want more tests on people and the companies will wish to keep the amount of expensive testing to a minimum.

If we are to have safer and more effective drugs, we must attempt to resolve these conflicts.

Note

I have not yet mastered non-sexist language. Therefore, man throughout is taken to mean a member of species homo sapiens, unless the context implies male adult. 'Animal' is taken to mean a living, sensate organism other than homo sapiens, unless the context is clearly inclusive.

References and Further Reading

Beauchamp, T. L. and Childress, J. F., *Principles of Biomedical Ethics* (Oxford: Oxford University Press, 1983).

BMA/Pharmaceutical Society. *British National Formulary* (11).

British Medical Association. *The Handbook of Medical Ethics* (London: BMA, 1984).

Duncan, A. S., Dunstan, G. R., and Welborne, R. B., *Dictionary of Medical Ethics* (London: Darton, Longman and Todd, 1981).

Duncan, A. S. (ed.) *Monthly Index of Medical Specialities*, January 1986.

Dunstan, G. R. and Seller, M. J. (eds), *Consent in Medicine* (King Edward's Hospital Fund, London, 1983).

Faulder, Carolyn, *Whose body is it?* (London: Virago Press, 1985).

Frey, R. G., *Interests and Rights* (Oxford: Clarendon Press, 1980).

Illich, I., *Limits to Medicine* (Harmondsworth: Penguin, 1977).

Kennedy, I., *The Unmmasking of Medicine* (London: Paladin, 1983).

Mason, J. K. and McCall Smith, R. A., *Law and Medical Ethics* (Butterworth, 1983).

Phillips, M. and Dawson, J., *Doctors Dilemmas* (Brighton: Harvester Press, 1985).

Singer, Peter, *In Defence of Animals* (Oxford: Blackwell, 1985).

Singer, Peter, *Animal Liberation* (Cape, 1977).

The Holy Bible (King James Version) esp. Genesis I, and Matthew 8.

11 Informed Consent

Peter Beck

'The Physician is the servant of the art.'

Hippocrates: *Epidemics*, I xi 1, 165.

Viewed from an historical perspective, the notion of 'informed consent' as a part of the relationship between physicians and patients is a 'johnny-come-lately'. Although it may appear self-evident that the obligations or duties of physicians and the rights or claims of patients are mutually implicatory, the directions and weights of these implications have been little considered before the present century. Whilst philosophers may have recognised a 'logical correlativity of rights and obligations' in general terms, such concepts have been applied historically in, at best, an asymmetrical way to the relations of patients and their doctors.

For example, although in the Hippocratic corpus (especially in the Oath) one finds descriptions of both physician and patient 'rights', there is little which concerns the concepts of consent – or even truth-telling. The main concerns for the physician relate firstly to the profession (not the patient) in requiring loyalty and respect for their teachers (and their offspring!) and a requirement to teach, though only to a 'chosen few'; towards patients a duty to the sick in terms of benefit is implied and, at most, an effort to avoid treatment which might be deleterious is required. Avoidance of exploitation of the 'special relationship', especially in terms of intimacies, is defined as is the demand to maintain confidentiality.

The corpus recognises three main components in what Engelhardt has termed 'this fabric of interests' – namely the disease, the patient and the physician – and goes on to define their relationship thus: 'The art has three factors, the disease, the patient, the physician. The physician is the servant of the art' (i.e. the profession). 'The patient must co-operate with the physician in combating the disease' (Hippocrates, *Epidemics*).

This paternalistic emphasis has persisted certainly well into the nineteenth century and in many areas persists today. In the early attempts to define Codes of Medical Ethics (e.g. American Medical Association, 1847) there is still no hint of modern conceptions of patients' rights or of physical obligations in allowing any input from the patient into the equation. The main requirements for the physician were still directed towards giving adequate care and maintaining confidentiality, but specifically forbade the giving of 'gloomy prognoses' – especially not informing patients of impending demise. Similarly patients were to tell all, avoid unqualified persons and submit unquestioningly to the orders of their physicians.

Clearly a relation has always existed between the duties of physicians and the rights of their patients, but equally clearly this has always been an unequal relationship. Perhaps there is some degree of inevitability in this. While the final enemy, death, is never ultimately defeated by the physician he is nevertheless usually in a more advantageous posture than his patient, who needs must seek his aid because he is ill. While the physicians' aim to 'cure sometimes, to care always' will be readily accepted by the patient, the patient's desire for these objectives has usually (at least until recent years) meant that he was willing to forego at least some of his rights (e.g. to freedom, privacy in achieving his desired aim).

As patients' perceptions of this relationship have increasingly involved them in notions of contract, however, patients' 'rights', in terms of claims on this contract, have become more vocalised. Recognition by patients of the positive rights of physicians to offer care, confidentiality etc. have been extended to the recognition of negative rights of refraining from impinging their freedom – e.g. by deception or other paternalistic actions. Similarly their own rights have been perceived as 'prima facie'; their right to 'health care' in terms of justice; their right to accept or refuse treatment in terms of autonomy, from a deontological perspective (though a [probably much weaker] utilitarian justification for such a patients' rights perspective is also definable).

Such desires of patients for care on their own terms (whatever their philosophical basis) have inevitably led to the concept of the requirement for consent of patients for treatment – a considerable departure from the historical situation outlined above. Perhaps because of the slowness of the medical profession to come to terms with this 'sea-change' in public expectations much of the categorisation and implementation of the change in terms of medical practice in therapeutic areas (i.e. 'caring for sick people') has arisen from case law. Equally the impact on medical research has been more reflected in codes of practice arising especially from the appalling realization of what had occurred under this guise in the Nazi camps (namely the Nuremberg Code and the Declaration of Helsinki). I propose therefore, at least in part, to look at the therapeutic and research aspects of consent separately.

Before doing so, however, further consideration must be given to the purpose or function of consent and to the justifications for it. Capron[1] has identified several functions:

1. The promotion of individual autonomy.
2. The protection of patients and subjects.
3. The avoidance of fraud and duress.
4. The encouragement of self-scrutiny by medical professionals.
5. The promotion of rational decisions.
6. The involvement of the public (in promoting autonomy as a general social value and in controlling biomedical research).

When considering the above list I suggest that all the propositions could be encompassed in two positions, namely the protection of the patient/subject from harm and the protection of the autonomy of the patient. Whilst the protection from harm, deriving from principles of non-maleficience and beneficence, will be also enhanced by laws, e.g. against battery and negligence, they would still, presumably, allow a physician, for such laudatory utilitarian ends, to 'protect' his patient from 'unwise' choices, and I feel therefore that the justification for autonomy (i.e. a deontological position) is much stronger than from the utilitarian principles outlined above.

If therefore the concept of patient consent to treatment is justified by this respect for his autonomy, is the 'mere' acceptance of allowing consent enough? Especially in the light of the increasing complication and sophistication of modern medical practice, is 'consent' a meaningful concept without the necessary informational elements which surely must be necessary to validate it? Thus the concept of consent must surely be broadened to encompass what has been (hopefully!) termed informed consent. It is clear that such consent will have therefore both informational and consent elements. Perhaps underpinning both of them there must also be considered the concept of competence to consent: can an incompetent be truly said to possess autonomy, which was the justification for consent in the first place? Competence cannot be considered as a rigid condition; the context is variable, and persons may have limited competence, e.g. be able to dress, feed and talk – even drive! – but be incompetent in more contemplative functions. Competence may also be variable; the fluctuations of an illness may well dictate that. Whilst the majority of cases may readily be defined as competent or not (at a particular time) there will certainly always be 'grey areas' and borderline cases and the standard for determining competence will be necessarily empirical and therefore liable to be value-laden. The unconscious or hopelessly demented will be clearly incompetent, but what of patients with (possibly remitting-relapsing) psychiatric illness? What of children? Separate rules will be necessary to attempt to preserve the 'potential' for autonomy for these patients in terms of consenting to treatment – and especially research - and the whole area of proxy-consent will clearly be relevant, but space does not permit a fuller exploration of this most important area in this essay (at least at this point!)

From considering competence as a presupposition for the concept of informed consent I shall return to the information elements of it. These must encompass not only the disclosure of information but its comprehension and could also legitimately be taken to include the area of truth-telling – which surely is a presupposition for the informational element of consent.

As hinted at early in the historical comments on consent, the need for truth-telling in doctor-patient relations is notable for its absence in historical codes. It may be questioned whether truth-telling is encompassed in a single duty of veracity or whether there are moral differences in direct lying, deception, non or partial disclosure (or using contemporary phraseology, 'being economical with the truth'). It could be argued that all of these violate patients' 'prima facie' rights (and if these encompass, in Mill's terms, 'duties of perfect obligation' – i.e. including correlative rights – as well as physicians' obligations). However a physician may argue that an infringement (violation) of patients' rights may, in certain circumstances, be justified, and that in these circumstances the principles of beneficence/non-maleficence could outweigh the patients' autonomy. For example, I may deem it justifiable to adopt a policy of intentional non-disclosure of the very likely bad prognosis of a severe coronary thrombosis to a patient so stricken and just admitted to my coronary care unit – on the grounds that to be gratuitously presented with such information at such a time would tend towards the production of a 'self-fulfilling prophecy' by increasing the patient's anxiety and distress at a time when all the medical evidence dictates a requirement to reduce them, in an attempt to improve the prognosis and save the patient's life. (The particular requirements for full disclosure of information in relation to both therapeutic and non-therapeutic research will be considered later in that context).

In general the standards for disclosure of information in the therapeutic context have derived considerably from case law and perhaps not surprisingly therefore ambiguities persist and the 'ground rules' are not unequivocably established and agreed. The most time-honoured (and still most prevalent) standard in both the UK and USA (1986) is still the 'professional practice' standard, although the second, the reasonable person standard appears to be emerging gradually as an acceptable legal criterion, though again some would modify this with a 'subjective' element.

The professional practice standard requires disclosure of information – particularly in relation to possible risks associated with a course of treatment as are consistent with the practice of the local medical community. Clearly this is a very paternalistic view emanating from the conviction that the doctor (as a representative of the profession) will always act in the best interests of his patient. The most telling argument against this must surely be that it undermines the autonomy of the patient – though other arguments, such as the difficulty in getting a group of doctors (especially surgeons!) to agree on 'standard practice' and the likelihood of such a policy 'enshrining bad practice merely because it is prevalent', also carry weight.

The reasonable person standard does attempt to go some way to redressing these arguments in that it gives greater weight to the patients' autonomy than to utilitarian aims of beneficence. Problems do arise with this standard also however, especially in terms of definition of the hypothetical 'reasonable person' and in defining their perceived views on, for example, acceptable risks. There are also problems in defining whether a known risk is 'material' or not, especially when related merely to the hypothetical reasonable person, rather than to the actual patient involved. This has led to some attempts to 'personalise' this standard to take account of the inevitably differing individual needs for information (in terms of complexity etc., and relating to a particular patient's problems, e.g. past medical history, special risk factors, etc.). Problems will arise in terms of defining how far it would be reasonable for a physician to go in determining (i.e. gaining enough information) a patient's 'tailor-made' informational needs. But from the moral (purely legal) point of view I feel that some combination of the reasonable person standard and an individualised element – which would give enough information to allow an informed decision to be made without regard to the eventual outcome – would be best: autonomy should still outweigh utilitarian considerations in attempting to provide the best informational elements for the informed consent decision to be made.

As well as merely ensuring adequate information there is also a need for adequate comprehension of the information before consent can be said to be really informed. One could argue that (for both doctor and patient) the concept of 'fully informed' is a myth. But in order for the consent to be valid, the necessary information – defined in terms of the standards above presupposing competence – must also be understood. This is a difficult area, not the least in terms of trying to assess whether comprehension has occurred or not. Many studies aimed at assessing levels of comprehension in patients who have been given information about their conditions have produced very disappointing results in terms of knowledge apparently acquired, or at least appreciated: appreciation does not necessarily equate with acceptance of information either, and some element of denial, especially with 'bad news', is undoubtedly common.

With this background of attempting to encompass the 'informational' elements of informed consent, consideration must also be given to the element of consent itself. As noted above, for the consent to be valid there is a presupposition of competence. The consent, however, must be voluntary to achieve validity. This infers that the consent is given without coercion – either overt or covert – and attempts to eliminate any unjustifiable ('controlling') influences. Clearly there will be a spectrum of influence on any decision and it would be impossible to control them all – or even to recognise them all. Coercion and influences can be very overt, e.g. brutality (Nazi doctors), financial (especially in non-therapeutic research), etc., but can also be much more subtle, e.g. hidden (from the doctors) family pressures, desire to please, etc. While the concept of fully voluntary choice is probably unattainable, attempts should certainly be made to exclude (especially 'controlling') influences on the basis (again) of respect for the patient's autonomy. The physician must never forget that in practical terms the doctor-patient interface is rarely value-free. Patients' perceptions of themselves in relation to their doctor are often inherently subservient and dependent, and what seems to the physician to be a mixture of disbursement of information 'shading' into rational persuasion may in reality 'shade' into compliance to perceived authority, which is certainly less than voluntary. Looked at from the point of view of moral principles and philosophical medical ethics, many of these decisions may appear to be relatively clear cut; in clinical practice, with individual patients with their particular problems, the distinctions can easily become blurred and the perceived clarity clouded.

The other large area where concern for informed consent is paramount is, of course, in medical research. The atrocities performed under this heading in Nazi Germany led directly to the Nuremberg Code, the first paragraph of which stated: 'The voluntary consent of the human subject is absolutely essential.' The whole concept of medical research on individuals raises basic moral problems. It is difficult to reconcile the Declaration of Geneva's statement: 'the health of my patient shall be my first concern' with doing experiments, however laudable their aim, in order to hopefully produce benefit for other, hypothetical 'future' patients. Some sort of balance has to be struck between a totally strict, all-encompassing regard for the autonomy of an individual patient and such possible utilitarian benefits to allow any medical research to occur.

This is much easier to achieve in relation to 'research' on an individual which may well produce benefit for the patient in their particular illness – so-called 'therapeutic' research, but much more difficult when the research is 'non-therapeutic' from that patient's point of view.

The Declaration of Helsinki (1975) has attempted to encompass some of the middle ground here, making a case (necessarily utilitarian) for the need for research in order to achieve any medical progress, but defining the ground rules ('Basic Principles') with some care and making clear distinctions between clinical and non-therapeutic research. The need for informed consent is emphasised in this document, together with requests for full information and respect for 'concern for the interests of the subject' which 'must always prevail over the interests of science and society'. However even this stress on the subject's autonomy is weakened when the same document, in the section on clinical research, can state: 'If the doctor considers it essential not to obtain informed consent, the specific reasons for this proposal should be stated on the experimental protocol . . .'. Clearly the potential for moral dilemmas remains!

Such dilemmas have often been most apparent in the discussions on 'who' should be recruited into research (particularly non-therapeutic) studies. Hans Jonas,[2] for example, has stated that 'utter helplessness demands utter protection' (perhaps this is really a statement about competence), but moves to a more utilitarian position when he avers that patients should only be experimented on in relation to their own disease. Paul Ramsey[3] regards research as a joint adventure between patient and doctor – 'a voluntary association of free men in a common cause' – but I feel that the propensity of medical scientists towards unbalancing the adventure in their favour makes valid informed consent still totally necessary.

The need for fully informed consent is perhaps most needed – and most potentially vulnerable – in the area of controlled trials, especially when the subjects are randomised to a treatment protocol in a study which demands that neither patient alone ('single-blind') nor patient or doctor ('double-blind') knows the nature of the treatment. There is no doubt that the informational elements in obtaining valid consent in such studies may be difficult to put across, but this does not mean that they can be therefore avoided or 'judged'.

Some physicians have maintained very paternalistic views in this area, alleging that obtaining informed consent may, for example, 'be not in the patient's best interests' – as the patient may lose confidence in a doctor who admits he does not know which is the 'best' treatment – or even (heaven forbid!) make an 'unwise decision' and decline treatment! They often make the point that informed consent is not customary in 'ordinary clinical practice' in terms of all the details of treatment decisions. To this I would argue that doctors should be seeking informed consent much more often than they do in these 'ordinary' areas, and therefore 'a fortiori' must do so in research situations.

Although the Declaration of Helsinki makes a clear-cut distinction between clinical and non-therapeutic research, such distinctions are sometimes blurred. Even the Declaration allows that subjects may be healthy volunteers or patients 'for whom the experimental design is not related to the patient's illness'. As soon as any patients are used the consent element, in terms of it being truly voluntary (as discussed above) becomes potentially less autonomous. And even with volunteers, the possibility of covert coercion (e.g. by payments to impoverished students or use of prisoners or service personnel) is a very real one.

It is clear, therefore, that for all the reasons detailed earlier, valid informed consent, in terms of both the informational and consent elements (and with just as much, if not more, regard for competence) is as needful some would say more needful – in medical research as it is in medical practice as a whole.

'Informed consent enables us to say no as well as yes'.[4]

Notes

1. A. M. Capron, 'Informed Consent in Catastrophic Disease and Treatment', *University of Pennsylvania Law Review* (1974) vol. 123, pp. 364–76.
2. H. Jones, 'Philosophical Reflections on Experimenting with Human Subjects', in T. L Beauchamp and L. Walters, *Contemporary Issues in Bioethics* (Belmont: Wadsworth, 1982) pp. 524–32.
3. P. Ramsey, 'Consent as a Canon of Loyalty', in Beauchamp and Walters, ibid., pp. 532-5.
4. C. Faulder, *Whose Body is it?* (London: Virago, 1985).

References

Beauchamp, T. L. and Childress, J. F., *Principles of Biomedical Ethics* (Oxford: Oxford University Press, 1983).

Beauchamp, T. L. and Walters L., *Contemporary Issues in Bioethics* (Belmont: Wadsworth, 1982).

Faulder, Carolyn, *Whose Body is it?* (London: Virago, 1985).

12 Autonomy, Competence and Mental Disorders

Patrick Nash

Informed consent has emerged, perhaps uniquely, in the field of health care, as a particular quality of consent by a patient to a particular treatment or course of treatment. Assuming legal competence, it requires that a decision, made without force or duress, is founded on appropriate understanding of the nature of the treatment, its probable outcomes including side effects as well as benefits, and appreciation of alternative treatment modes.

While conceptually it is a simple concept, considerations of normal human psychology suggest that in absolute form it will not be easy to achieve in every patient–professional relationship. In addition for the conscientious practitioner these are the problems created by the interconnection of philosophical, legal, as well as clinical issues implicit in the concept. Despite that well recognised difficulty there is no perspective which is shared across the boundaries of the relevant disciplines to assist the practitioner in the resolution of problems at an operational level (Eth and Robb, 1986). The frustration experienced by the medical profession as a result may be seen in the literature where, not uncommonly, informed consent will be castigated as, for instance, 'a legalistic function' (Hamilton, 1983), or even as having no existence at all (Lafret, 1976).

Such a response may also have its root in the traditional commitment of the medical profession to 'beneficence' rather than to autonomy. It is only since the era of the Second World War that the profession has been obliged to come to terms in a real way with the moral principle of autonomy, from which the idea of informed consent is derived, although only in the last twenty years has it emerged in developed form (Hamilton, 1983).

The model of informed consent proposed by Lidz *et al.* (1984) is valuable for the clarity with which the components of the concept are set out and their internal cohesion demonstrated:

$$C + I \rightarrow U$$
$$U + V \rightarrow D$$

Competence (C): Patient must have the competence (a) in law to give consent; and (b) in fact to understand the information given.

Information (I): Patient must be given information about diagnosis, proposed treatment, positive and negative outcomes, and alternative treatment modes.

Understand (U): This will be assumed in a patient when appropriate competence and information are established.

Voluntariness (V): Patient must be free of coercion and duress.

Decision (D): Patient's choice finally must be his alone.

Such a model has the benefit of clarity, but is clearly 'rational-legal', and for that reason is not always useful in clinical practice when the obtaining of consent is part of an on-going patient-physician relationship.

Clearly the focus of informed consent is on the moral, legal and political independence of the individual, while beneficence, and the paternalism to which it gives rise in the doctor–patient relationship, focuses primarily on the needs of a patient as perceived finally by the physician. It is the conflict of these principles in health-care practice which gives rise to the frustration which can be experienced by both patient and practitioner in the clinical situation.

Clinical problems rather than philosophical differences will most often be advanced as being central in obtaining informed consent, but it is apparent both in discussion and from the extensive literature that problems exist at the philosophical level. There appears to be no acknowledgement from the medical profession particularly, although not exclusively, of the patient's autonomous nature as a person where that would seem to interfere with the expedient benevolence of the practitioner. Such views are implicit in much that is written about informed consent: '(informed consent) . . . destroys good patient care and paralyses the conscientious physician' (Lafret, 1976). Hamilton (1983), after detailing the problems of providing information to patients, describes the requirement for 'understanding' as 'the entry of nonsense', and asserts that attempts to make informed consent conform to 'lawyers' requirements' are 'best described as pathetic'.

However, it is of course the law rather than lawyers of which clinicians need to be aware of in the first instance, and undoubtedly the law regards consent from competent adults as a significant element in human rights, nationally and internationally (see, for example, United Nations Declaration, European Convention, Helsinki Agreement). D'Entreves (1976) proposes that autonomy can be seen as a derivative of a right to liberty as a natural right, or, as Veatch maintains (1981), 'a rational necessity for the foundation of a moral system and an essential part of the social covenant'. Certainly a change can be described over centuries from the emphasis on individualism derived from a natural law ontology to the philosophical concept of autonomy and its recognition as a prerequisite in a moral system.

The work of Kant (Lindley, 1986) can be seen as a link between the traditional Chartian, natural law, position and rapidly developing secular philosophies of the seventeenth century. What Kant regarded as a categorical moral requirement was the exercise of rationality and will by each individual so that his life and relationships with others are guided by principled reasons which at least he must freely will where he is not the author of them. That free exercise of reason and will for Kant is the hallmark of autonomy, itself a condition to be presumed in others, and marking out the human being as a master of choices and thus a being of unconditional worth, never to be treated as a means, always as an end (Lindley, 1986). That principle of autonomy allows Kant to elaborate his proposition that a moral law of conduct must be such that its author would willingly have it apply universally including to himself, confident that its impact will enhance rather than diminish the autonomy of all.

Whereas the focus of morality in Kant is in reason and will, that of J. S. Mill is on action, his principle being that in self regarding actions man must be free to the point where the freedom of another is impinged. In contrast to Kant, Mill's justification is social and utilitarian rather than individual and deontological. He asserts that the freedom of the individual to exercise his talents without interference will enhance overall creativity and finally tend to maximise benefit for all. Despite the differing premises of Kant and Mill, their conclusions finally lead to autonomy enhancing behaviour. However neither approach is accepted without challenge.

A particular weakness in Kant's position is perhaps his assumption of the possibility of intellect and will freely exercised in beings whose physiology will inevitably effect both to a degree unknown to the individual (Lindley, 1986). The element of contradiction implicit in Mill's position has been mentioned above, and certainly the logic of the traditional utilitarian position would always subject the individual to the 'greater good' of society. However some utilitarian philosophers would continue to assert the value of the retention by the individual of some areas of autonomous decision making. The justification advanced by Dasgupta (1982), for instance, is based on the use of information which can be known uniquely only by the individual in enhancing decision-making in the market economy. His principle is particularly interesting in that it would appear to apply appropriately in the health-care situation where much of the subjective information bearing on a treatment decision is unquestionably unique to the patient (particularly affective and social data) and may be such as to defeat any attempt by the patient to communicate it to the professional, for reasons of confidentiality, perhaps anxiety or embarrassment, and certainly in many cases because of problems in communication and language (see the work of Bernstein, 1971, on language and social class.)

Despite unresolved philosophical difficulties there does exist in liberal democratic societies, of which health-care professionals form a part, a consensus that autonomy can be rationally defined as a prerequisite of moral action. It is interesting to note, however, as Beauchamp and Childress (1983) point out, that not all autonomous action will be moral, and Foot (1978) commenting on Nietzsche points to the rejection of all social morality which he would require a priori from the 'higher' man. This rejection of authority is not required for autonomy by philosophers generally where, for instance, it operates in the interest of the autonomy of others (Mill), or is accepted for principled reasons (Kant).

In that connection Hayek's (1960) discussion of the meaning of the word 'freedom' is particularly helpful. He offers 'independence of the arbitrary will of another' as the primary meaning, but suggests that one should distinguish further: (a) political freedom, (b) inner, or metaphysical freedom, and (c) liberty. The last two are of particular value in considering informed consent in psychiatry because both inner freedom, 'extent to which a person is guided in his actions by his own considered will rather than by emotion or by moral or intellectual weakness', and liberty, i.e. 'the ability to do what the individual wishes', may be significantly infringed, the first by the disorder and its treatment, the second in many cases by the requirements of the law.

Psychiatry, perhaps more than other areas of medical practice, has been subject to pressures engendered by increasing emphasis on patient autonomy which emerged following revelations of medical malpractice in wartime Nazi Germany. Developing from that period advances in the science and technology of medicine were accompanied by heightened sensitivity individually and politically to issues of personal freedom and civil liberty, and in the United States and Canada increasingly willingness by the Courts to penalise doctors whose patients suffered damage, the likelihood of which had not been disclosed to them.

In addition over the last twenty years there developed on both sides of the Atlantic a degree of disillusionment with science and authority which can be seen as contributing to the sustained attack on psychiatry, both from within (see, for example, Szasz, Laing and generally the 'Italian Movement'), and in the UK, externally, from the media and public opinion, which very largely eroded traditional psychiatric powers of coercion in admission, restraint and treatment.

Whether the anti-authoritarian thinking which is involved to some degree in such onslaughts would be included among the 'important reasons' which for Beauchamp and Childress (1983) may justifiably override autonomy is open to question, but certainly the prevention of harm to others would be such a reason, and psychiatrists would assert it as central to the traditional role which has been theirs. Equally it could be asserted that by psychiatric definition (at least), their patients may not have achieved autonomy, for instance the psychopath, or have temporarily lost it, for instance the psychotic. That diminution of rationality and/or volition implicit in such a condition would indicate some loss of autonomy may be deduced for Kant from the emphasis on these elements in his work.

For Mill, also, autonomy is not absolute in all. He exempted the young, the mentally disordered and primitive peoples, and though attitudes have developed since with reference to children (see, for instance, DHSS, 'Bridges over Troubled Waters', 1986) and differently ordered societies, his position overall on this issue (Bloch and Chodoff, 1984) would appear to lend support to psychiatric intervention.

However although psychiatry would appear, superficially at least, to have both the law (MHA, 1983) and philosophy on its side, there remains the fundamental difficulty raised by the absence of consensus, or of empirical data, as to what mental disorder is, or indeed if it exists at all or is merely a myth created and sustained by psychiatrists (Szasz, 1971). Equally, the orthodox psychiatric view requires that the behaviours alleged to support a diagnosis of mental disorder are in fact irrational rather than unusual (Lindley, 1986) and may justifiably be used to evidence loss of Hayek's 'inner or metaphysical freedom' to the point where autonomy may safely be said to be either diminished or absent.

Similar problems exist with attempts to assert 'dangerousness' as justification for interference with freedom of action. Psychiatrists are known as very poor predictors of dangerousness in their patients (Gostin, 1976), and if 'danger to self' is used as ethical justification it would not satisfy Mill's criteria and, frequently accompanied by apparent rationality and sound personality function, could not meet the requirements of a Kantian view.

One result of the emergence of informed consent as a focus for public concern in medicine has been a heightening of awareness generally to the issue of autonomy and an equivalent development in the justification of the traditional medical position. Defences vary from mere assertion of orthodox medical values (e.g. Hamilton, 1983) to more considered argument (Komrad 1983; and in psychiatry, Chodoff, 1984), but still from within the medical context.

McIntyre (1975) offers an explanation for this adherence to the orthodox medical view. He suggests that the disappearance from society of the once settled morality of Christianity and its replacement with liberal and secular pluralism has left us 'resourceless' in the face of moral problems. Therefore, in his view, doctors will understandably rely on what he sees as the 'certainties' of what is an essentially paternalistic morality. In psychiatry there is evidence of a stronger certainty amounting to moral imperialism, in which the values of psychiatry are made to eradicate the concepts of ethics and law from doctor–patient relations by a process of reduction. Moore (1984) explores this subtle process in some detail, suggesting that where illness is the primary focus, then moral terms are minimised and finally eradicated as being inapplicable to the behaviours to which they would in other relationships apply. Certainly, evidence of this process is common in clinical practice where judgements of 'good' and 'bad' with reference to behaviour in certain patients are absent, and medical evaluations of illness and 'normality' are offered as more appropriate.

The anti-psychiatry movement represents a major backlash from within against such a 'psychiatrisation of life' (refer Szasz, and Laing), and the Italian Movement (Tranchina, 1981) evidences massive rejection of the psychiatrisation process in a society which also helped to legitimise coercion as a response to mental disorder. The wish by some practitioners to spread psychiatric values beyond patients is clear in the literature, where from time to time both law and philosophy come under fire when seen to advocate patient autonomy and informed consent. Hamilton (1983) would have the lawyers accept the wisdom of the 'wise men' of psychiatry on informed consent, and Wood (1982) is prepared to reduce ethical debate first to practicalities, then to pragmatism. In advocating such a view Wood is simply reflecting the act utilitarianism position widely held in medicine (Eth and Robb, 1986). Wood, like many practitioners appears not to consider the accompanying danger that it can lead on to opportunism and expediency, neither ethical nor professional, and so reinforce the anxieties of the public and add to the ongoing critique of psychiatry.

On the other hand, it can be shown that both patients and society have contributed to the psychiatric value system. Over many years psychiatry has offered to innumerable unhappy people relief from guilt and responsibility, and in order to succeed it has required both individual and societal acquiescence in its transmutation of 'bad' to 'sick'. Society responded with legislation permitting the psychiatrist alone to decide, in all except criminal cases, where on that spectrum an individual's deviant behaviour should be seen to lie. Patients for the most part have accepted such evaluations and their own minimisation as 'sick', in exchange for relief from personal unhappiness and responsibility. It can be seen that implicit in acceptance of such a subordinate role is the marginalisation of concepts like autonomy and informed consent, which are founded on personal responsibility for the self.

In professional practice, where the existence of mental disorder is accepted by both doctor and patient, the problems raised for psychiatrists in obtaining informed consent are often greater than in other areas of medicine. The psychiatrist is faced with a patient whose autonomy is already constrained internally by his pathology and whose treatment may require that it be further reduced temporarily or permanently. In addition the patient may be one whose freedom has been legally removed, or if informal, may be equally restricted by his situation within a basically coercive system (Hoggett, 1984).

These two practical realities will affect either the 'understanding' or 'voluntary' elements in informed consent, and they exist in addition to any difficulties imposed by intelligence, education, or the effects of the 'special dimension of anguish' (Komrad, 1983) which may create difficulty in any medical specialty. That phenomenon, for Komrad, allied to the knowledge gap between patient and professional, so reduces patient autonomy a priori that the benevolent paternalism of medicine operates not to reduce it further, but in fact to restore it, and the doctor emerges as 'champion of autonomy'. A difficulty with Komrad's interesting argument is his assumption of the moral conscientiousness of physicians generally; his belief that this paternalism will be wise and benevolent is in marked contrast to that of Chodoff (1984).

As a psychiatrist, having argued the case for paternalism in involuntary admission and treatment, he asserts: 'the paternalism I espouse should not be presumed to be wise and benevolent, rather, chastened and self critical, it should be willing to submit to strong safeguards against abuse.' Such a view recognises that wisdom may exist beyond the borders of medicine, and would acknowledge society's attempts through parliament (MHA, 1983) to balance the patient's loss of freedom of action with some continuing control on treatment decisions. The statutory system designed to achieve that goal is not unlike in its effects the 'weak paternalism' described by Feinberg (1974), 'to prevent self-regarding conduct only when it is substantially non-voluntary, or, when temporary intervention is required to establish whether it is voluntary or not'.

In the legislation, compulsory treatment is taken as a separate issue from compulsory admission. Treatments are divided into those which may never be given without consent, and those which in some circumstances may be. For the former, third parties are involved to validate consent and provide supporting medical opinion; in the latter case, in the absence of consent, a second medical opinion must be obtained if the treatment is to proceed. Unfortunately the effect of these requirements despite their estimable intent is to create a series of ethical double-binds for the psychiatrist. Three examples are offered as illustration.

(1) A compulsory patient may be treated with drugs for a period of three months, without his consent, after which time the safeguards outlined above will apply (MHA 1983, S58). For the psychiatrist, while the legislation exempts him from legal obligation to obtain the consent, the drugs he may wish to use to restore what Hayek terms 'inner autonomy' may affect volition in such a way that inner autonomy may be affected to the point that the patient is unlikely to resist suggestions for treatment when eventually in a legal position to do so.

(2) Taylor (1983) raises the question of whether refusal of ECT for severe depression can ever be a 'competent' decision, given that such a disorder must inevitably affect judgement to some extent, and that the treatment, despite controversy, is recognised by the profession as specific and effective? Legally, absence of consent may be disregarded when a second medical opinion is obtained, but the ethical problem for the clinician remains.

(3) For some treatments, whether the patient is informal or compulsory, the legislation requires validated, real consent, and a supporting medical opinion (MHA 1983, S56(1) and (2), and S57). The intention is clearly to promote autonomy and eradicate both duress and coercion (especially in compulsory patients) from the consent process. The interesting ethical situation which this gives rise to is the exercise of strong state paternalism which reduces not only professional autonomy but also that of the patient who is informal. In that case consent is subject to mandatory third-party scrutiny, and a preferred treatment choice made conditional on third-party agreement.

Such examples would support the assertion that informed consent in psychiatry presents particular problems, over and above those normally to be found in medicine. The psychiatrist and those working with him must deal with the moral issues involved, and also with legislative requirements which, while enhancing patient autonomy, put the practitioner in a double-bind situation.

The central problems are the constraints on 'inner' freedom which are implicit in the concept of mental disorder and the demands of mental health legislation which go beyond the common law. Such a view will certainly suggest the aptness of Sider and Clements' assertion (1982) that standard legal and ethical models of informed consent are incomplete because they assume a 'linear' process between rational autonomous parties and an existential focus on a 'momentary point' of decision. Psychiatry requires, in contrast, what they term a 'recursive and dialogical' model in which informed consent cannot be abstracted from the physician–patient relationship. Finally the decision will be consensual, but time and non-consenting intervention will be required in many instances if inner freedom is to be restored to the point at which dialogue can be meaningful (see also Somerville, 1986, re psycho-geriatrics). Psychiatry requires that attention be given to non-rational factors like sensitivity and bonding which do not fit easily into the totally rational models, e.g. Lidz *et al.*

However the outright rejection of the legal/philosophical perspective has the greater danger perhaps of allowing psychiatrists to operative exclusively within a medical-psychiatric value system lacking a sound philosophical base, and reinforcing attitudes to 'non-medical' ethics which reduce them to hypothetical rather than categorical systems (see Moore, 1984; Foot, 1976), so that psychiatry becomes increasingly the application of exclusively professional generalisations (Engelhardt, 1975).

It is doubtful if fully satisfactory solutions can ever be found to the difficulties faced by the conscientious moral practitioner. However it is certain that his willingness to recognise them as difficulties is to be preferred to 'solutions' of many radical polemicists whose exclusive focus on autonomy and liberty appears to disregard the principles of beneficence and non-maleficence, inevitably adding to the unhappiness of many mentally disordered people (Sherlock, 1986).

Although ready answers cannot be found to the conceptual and philosophical problems raised by informed consent, it may be that they will become less acute as mandatory safeguards on autonomy are better tolerated by the profession while the present policy of community treatment is pursued. Within the community the coercive effects of institutional psychiatry do not apply, the patient will often feel the support of his social network, and dialogue between professional and patient is more likely to lead to consensus. The psychiatrist is also less constrained by the legislation and can approach the resolution of such problems on the basis of professionalism and ethics, within the requirements of common law, rather than in the context of the hospital and compulsory detention where he is coerced by legal requirements which make his professionalism and ethical position secondary.

In the situation of rapid social and technological change which will continue to affect medicine and psychiatry, Clouser's contention (1975) that 'it is not as though medical ethics were a recent invention . . . it is the "old ethics" trying to find its way around in new and puzzling circumstances' may be of value.

References

Beauchamp, T. L. and Childress, J. F., *Principles of Biomedical Ethics* (New York: Oxford University Press, 1983).

Bernstein, B., *Class, Codes and Control, VI* (London: Routledge, Kegan Paul, 1971).

Bloch, S. and Chodoff, P. (eds), *Psychiatric Ethics* (Oxford: Oxford University Press, 1984).

Chodoff, P. 'Involuntary Hospitalisation of M.I. as a Moral Issue', *American Journal of Psychiatry* (1984) vol. 141, no. 3, pp. 384–9.

Clouser, D.,'Medical Ethics: Uses, Abuses, Limitations', *New England Journal of Medicine* (1979) vol. 293, pp. 384–8.

Dasgupta, P., 'Utilitarianism, Information and Rights', in A. Sen and B. Williams (eds), *Utilitarianism and Beyond* (London: Cambridge University, Press 1982).

D'Entreres, A. P., *Natural Law* (London: Hutchinson University Library, 1976).

DHSS, *Bridges Over Troubled Waters* (London: HMSO 1986).

Engelhardt, H., Tristram and Spicker, S. F., *Evaluation and Explanation in Bio-medical Sciences* (Utrecht: D. Reidel Publishing Co., 1975).

Eth, S. and Robb, J., 'Informed Consent: the Problem', in D. K. Kentsmith, S. A. Salladay and P.A. Maya (eds), *Ethics in Mental Health Practice* (London: Grune and Stratten, 1986).

Feinberg, J., 'Legal Paternalism', Com. Jrn. Philosophy (1974), vol. 1, pp. 113–16, in Kentsmiths *et al.* (1986).

Foot, P., *Virtues and Vices* (London: Basil Blackwell, 1978).

Gostin, L., 'A Human Condition' VII. *MIND* London (1976).

Hamilton, M., 'On Informed Consent', *British Journal of Psychology* (1983) vol. 143, pp. 416–18.

Hayek, F. A., *The Constitution of Liberty* (London: Routledge, Kegan Paul, 1960).

Hoggett, B., *Mental Health Law*, 2nd edn. (London: Sweet and Maxwell, 1984).

Kentsmith, K., Salladay, S. A. and Miya, P. A. (eds), *Ethics in Mental Health Practice* (London: Grune and Stratten, 1986).

Komrad, M. S., 'Defence of Medical Paternalism', *Journal of Medical Ethics* (1983), vol. 9, pp. 38–44.

Lafret, E. G., 'Fiction of Informed Consent', *Journal of the American Medical Association* (1976), vol. 235, pp. 1579–85.

Lindley, R., *Autonomy* (London: Macmillan, 1986).

Lidz, C. W., *Informed Consent* (London: Guildford Press, 1984).

McIntyre, J., 'How Virtues becomes Vices', in Englehardt (1975).
Moore, M. S., *Law and Psychiatry* (London: Cambridge University Press, 1984).
Sen A. and Williams, B., *Utilitarianism and Beyond* (London: Cambridge University Press, 1982).
Sherlock, R. 'My Brother's Keeper?' in Kentsmith *et al.* (1986).
Sider, R. and Clements, C., 'Psychiatry's Contribution to Medical Ethics Education', *American Journal of Psychology* (1982), vol. 139, no. 4, pp. 498–501.
Siegler, M., quoted in Komrad (1983), p. 40.
Somerville, M. A., 'Legal and Ethical Aspects of Decision-Making for Aged Persons', in Kentsmith *et al.* (eds) (1986).
Szasz, M. T., *The Manufacture of Madness* (London: Routledge, Kegan Paul, 1971).
Taylor, P. J., 'Consent, Competency and ECT', *Journal of Medical Ethics* (1983) vol. 9, pp. 146–51.
Tranchina, P. *et al.*, 'New Legislation in Italian Psychiatry', *International Journal of Law and Psychiatry*, vol. 4, pp. 181–90.
Veatch, R. M., *A Theory of Medical Ethics* (New York: Basic Books, 1981).
Wood, J. C., 'Impact of Legal Modes of Thought on the Practice of Psychiatry', *British Journal of Psychiatry* (1982), vol. 14, pp. 551–63.

13 Compulsory Care

Richard Bentall

In recent years it has been a matter of some concern to psychiatrists and others in the West that political dissidents in the Soviet Union have been diagnosed as mentally ill and have been involuntarily confined to psychiatric hospitals for treatment. It has thus been argued that Soviet psychiatrists have been guilty of the misuse of their psychiatric powers for political ends, usually on the grounds that the dissidents confined to hospital are in fact mentally well. In this paper it is shown that Western commentators cannot be complacent about their ability to defend this position because: (a) the concept of mental illness is unclear; (b) even so far as the concept of mental illness can be made clear it may be difficult to determine whether particular individuals – either in the West or the East – are mentally ill or mentally well; (c) in any case, illness qua illness cannot be a justification for compulsory treatment. It is suggested that there may be grounds for the compulsory treatment of individuals who lack rational autonomy, so long as rational autonomy is defined in a particular way. However, it is unlikely that this concept can be used to distinguish between the practices of Soviet and Western psychiatrists because many patients diagnosed as severely mentally ill may be able to demonstrate rational autonomy. An implication of this argument is that, as in the Soviet Union, much of psychiatric practice in the West amounts to the state-licensed control of deviance.

I

Imagine the following scenario: It is a meeting of the World Psychiatric Association. Psychiatrists from all over the world have gathered to exchange ideas and opinions about psychiatric research and practice. One of the highlights of the conference is a symposium on the ethics of involuntary hospitalisation in which psychiatrists from socialist countries are to confront psychiatrists from the freedom loving democracies of the West. Representing the western democracies is a consultant psychotherapist from Great Britain, Dr Western Block (known as 'West' to his friends) from Cambridgeshire. Representing the communist countries is Dr Eastern Block (known as 'East' to his comrades), a consultant psychiatrist working for the KGB in Moscow. Both psychiatrists have agreed to open the symposium by describing cases of involuntary psychiatric hospitalisation that typify psychiatric practice under their respective political regimes. First, it is West's turn.

West walks to the front of the conference room. He is a neatly but casually dressed man with warm blue eyes. He begins his talk with a smile. His case study can be summarised as follows: One night in the depths of winter he is summoned by a family doctor who is deeply concerned about the mental health of a patient, a young woman (Mrs A) who only two months previously has given birth to her first child. Twenty minutes later, West arrives at Mrs A's house to find, together with Mrs A, the doctor, Mrs A's husband, their young child, and her husband's two parents. It is immediately apparent that Mrs A is severely distressed. The doctor reports that Mrs A has spent most of the evening running from house to house in the neighbourhood pleading for help from her neighbours. However, she has been unable to say what kind of help she wants. When West tries to interview her all she can offer is a few vague comments to the effect that she feels persecuted by unspecified 'them'. Mr A also proves to be too agitated to give a coherent account of what has happened, but does hint that he suspects that his wife has been having a long-standing affair, that he himself is almost certainly infertile, and that he therefore has the strongest suspicions that he is not the natural father of the child. Fortunately, Mr A's parents appear to be in better command of their senses. They tell West that they were called from their home earlier in the evening by their son, that they are very worried for the health and safety of their son, their daughter-in-law and their grandchild, and that they are willing to do whatever they can to help. On the basis of the available evidence West reaches the following tentative conclusions: that Mrs A is suffering from a severe post-natal depression and that she may be a risk to herself and to her child. Accordingly, West asks Mr A's parents to look after the child and has Mrs A hospitalised so that she can be carefully observed by trained psychiatric nurses. Because Mrs A is unwilling to leave her home it becomes necessary to have her admitted to hospital as an involuntary patient.[1]

West sits down to polite applause. Now East rises to speak. In contrast to West, East wears a shabby suit that looks at least one size too large. His eyes shift nervously from side to side as he talks. His case study can be summarised as follows: Late one night he is summoned from his bed by a KGB officer who has just raided a flat in a Moscow suburb. Twenty minutes later East arrives at the flat to find the officer, a junior policeman, and the occupants of the flat, Mr and Mrs Z. The KGB officer explains that Mr Z has long been under surveillance under suspicion of preaching anti-Soviet propaganda. One month previously Mr Z was dismissed from his job for economic sabotage (he tried to get his fellow workers to strike in demand for free trade unions). On searching the flat the officer and his comrade have found anti-Soviet literature printed by the government of the United States of America. When East attempts to interview Mr Z he is sullen, uncooperative and declines to answer East's questions except with the briefest 'yes' or 'no'. When East persists, however, Mr Z suddenly becomes angry and accuses East of persecuting him. Meanwhile, Mrs Z becomes more and more upset and finally breaks down in tears. East makes a provisional diagnosis (using the Moscow School of Psychiatry's diagnostic criteria) of 'sluggish schizophrenia'. The KGB officer and his comrade duly take Mr Z off to the Serbsky Institute of Forensic Psychiatry where he can be closely observed by highly qualified psychiatric staff.[2]

East sits down to stunned silence from the audience. Psychiatrists from the West sit with their mouths agape. Those from the East hide their heads in embarrassment, not having expected their colleague to deliver such a candid account of Soviet psychiatric practice. Suddenly, the silence is broken by West who stands up and, in a loud voice, accuses East of using psychiatry to the detriment of fundamental human rights. At West's words, pandemonium breaks out with western and eastern psychiatrists shouting abuse and condemnation at each other. The manager of the conference centre, hearing the commotion, takes a look in the conference room and immediately tells a junior to send for the police.

The conviction that psychiatrists from the Soviet Union and other eastern block countries have been using powers of hospital detention and compulsory treatment to suppress political dissent has been of considerable concern to western psychiatrists in recent years.[3] Behind this concern is (presumably) the belief that cases like that of Mrs A differ in important ways from those like that of Mr Z. But can any substance be given to this belief? Suppose that West and East were to calm down and to argue rationally about their differences? Is there anything that West could say to persuade East that the case of Mrs A is logically different from the case of Mr Z? In the remainder of this paper I hope to show that West (and by implication any western psychiatrist) cannot be complacent about his ability to do this.

II

What, then, would be West's first line of attack? It would probably be to argue that, whereas Mrs A suffered from a real form of 'mental illness', Mrs Z did not, so that in consequence West's decision to hospitalise Mrs A was a proper medical judgement whereas East's decision to detain Mr Z amounted to suppression of political dissent. Thus we are told by one western commentator that, 'since the late 1950s a small, but nevertheless significant, proportion of dissenters in the Soviet Union have been diagnosed, although mentally well, as suffering from such serious psychiatric conditions as schizophrenia and paranoid personality disorder'.[4] There would seem to be a number of hidden premises to this argument, namely (1a) that there is an objectively definable entity known as 'mental illness'; (1b) that in at least some cases of mental illness it is legitimate to deprive the sufferer of his autonomy and to force him to receive hospital treatment; and (1c) that unless someone is suffering from objectively defined mental illness it is wrong to force them to receive psychiatric treatment against their will.

The question of whether there really is such a thing as mental illness has been so extensively, but inconclusively, debated that it is with some hesitation that I raise this issue in the present context. However, the fact that it has been so extensively debated at the very least indicates that the existence of objectively definable mental illness cannot be taken for granted. Critics of the 'medical model' of insanity from both within and outside psychiatry have advanced a number of arguments. For example, the psychiatrist Thomas Szasz[5] has argued that, in the absence of demonstrable cerebral pathology, mental illness cannot qualify as 'illness' and that the diagnosis of mental illness therefore represents a form of value judgement qualitatively different from that involved in the diagnosis of physical illness. In a somewhat similar vein, the sociologist Thomas Scheff[6] has suggested that psychiatry is a method of social control used to label and contain certain types of social rule-breakers. On a quite different tack again, behavioural psychologists have claimed that abnormal behaviour is best understood and manipulated by the application of laws governing normal behaviour rather than by the use of medical concepts and treatment.[7] In contrast, defenders of traditional psychiatry argue that research shows that many forms of mental disorder are best understood in biological terms, and that there are certain recognisable syndromes consisting of meaningful clusters of symptoms which have certain predictable outcomes.[8]

It is not my purpose to resolve this dispute in the present context; I will attempt to show later that the question of the identity of mental disorder has no bearing on the present issue. However, it will be useful, at least in passing, to consider the tactics of the debate. Essentially, both sides compare criterion cases of mental illness (such as schizophrenia, the affective psychoses) with medical illnesses (such as diabetes, temporal lobe epilepsy), the proponents of the medical model claiming a series of family resemblances between the two sets of phenomena, the opponents of the medical model claiming that the differences are more convincing. Cast in this light, West's argument amounts to no more than the claim that the case of Mrs A has more in common with other medical conditions than has the case of Mr Z.

It is an open question whether West can be convincing in this respect. The aim of placing mental disorder within the scope of the concept of 'illness' is presumably to justify the application of medical concepts, research, treatments and technologies in these cases.[9] Not surprisingly, therefore, much of the debate about the concept of mental illness has focused on the identification of particular syndromes with particular (usually biological) causes, which lead to particular outcomes, and which respond to particular treatments.[10] Now it may be that the case of Mrs A corresponds with such a syndrome, although the particular context of her breakdown (her affair, her husband's impotence, his parents' concern about their 'ownership' of the baby) strongly suggests that a more appropriate parallel might be drawn with political disputes (for example, between nations arguing about territory or between unions seeking to control particular industries). But can West be sure that the case of Mr Z does not fit an illness model? Suppose that, following further investigation at the Serbsky Institute of Forensic Psychiatry it is discovered that Mr Z has long been a consumer of large doses of illicit amphetamine?[11] Suppose further, that on being weaned off his habit he develops a more tolerant attitude towards the government of his country?

This raises the question of how the case of Mrs A appears to East. One thing that East may do, in response to West's arguments, is to redescribe the case of Mrs A as a case of suppression of dissent. He might do this in order to argue either that Mrs A does not suffer from true mental illness, whereas Mr Z does or that all decisions to give compulsory treatment are ideological. A plausible account of the case of Mrs A might run as follows: Mr A and his parents feel that, if it becomes widely believed that Mrs A's child was not sired by her husband, they will lose any rights they have over the upbringing of the child. They have therefore (consciously or unconsciously) elected to maintain the existing family system by discrediting Mrs A's view of reality. Mrs A, feeling persecuted but unable to articulate this feeling (perhaps because she senses that others will doubt her sanity), has sought help from her neighbours but (especially as it is late at night and neighbours lack patience) has been unable to specify the help required. Meanwhile, Mr A and his parents have recruited West. When Mrs A tells West that she feels persecuted by 'them' she is expressing a real fear that her husband and his parents will take her child away from her. West, however, sides with Mr A and his parents and (perhaps unwittingly) has Mrs A locked away where she can no longer cause trouble.

How plausible this account seems will depend upon one's metapsychiatric theory. It certainly will not appeal to many psychiatrists in Europe or the United States, or even in the Soviet Union, who are generally biological in orientation and who tend to view what patients say when in a distressed state of mind as signs of disturbance rather than as meaningful communications.[12] Yet there is reason to believe that even the most psychotic utterances should not be dismissed so lightly. Certainly, the attempt to take psychotic communications seriously can be illuminating. Within the psychiatric literature Laing, in particular, has argued for the meaningfulness of psychotic speech.[13] Although Laing's views have generally been dismissed by prominent psychiatrists they have received some support from the experiences of at least some psychologists.[14] Laing has also made the case that psychotic patients are often the victims of persecutory family systems that elect the identified patients as insane in order to maintain the family status quo.[15] This latter view has, if anything, been even more vigorously rejected by the psychiatric establishment[16] but seems more credible in the light of recent developments in the family treatment of psychotic individuals.[17] Experimental psychology also gives some reason for believing that psychotic utterances may be meaningful. For example, the limited experimental literature on delusions suggests that they may be meaningful attributions[18] subject to change in the face of reasoned counter-argument.[19]

Of course, these considerations alone are not enough to knock down West's arguments against East. After all, it may in fact be the case that Mrs A's distress is mainly caused by a biochemical disturbance in her brain whereas Mr Z's is not (or vice versa). It might also be objected that the case of Mrs A is not representative of much of Western psychiatric practice. All that has been shown so far is that West ought not to be too hasty in criticising East given his relative lack of familiarity with East's cases, the limited scientific understanding of the causes of mental disorder, and the equivocal status of mental illness qua illness.

III

Whatever the merits of regarding particular examples of unusual behaviour as illness, there is an even more serious weakness in West's argument against East. This lies in the second hidden premise: that it is legitimate in at least some cases of mental illness to force someone to receive hospital treatment. Why should the diagnosis of mental illness, even if it could be made objectively, justify the removal of fundamental human rights? That it cannot be illness per se which provides this justification can be seen by considering the strongest possible defence that West could put against East's claim that Mrs A was not mentally ill.

Suppose West was to counter East by producing a mass of scientific evidence such that any reasonable observer would accept that Mrs A suffered from a genuine illness. For example, West might introduce a colleague, Dr Arthur Neurone, who has carried out a long series of research studies of people suffering with Mrs A's symptoms. Dr Neurone might report, for example, that in all cases so far studied of young women who develop paranoid symptoms in reaction to family stress following childbirth, a lesion has been detected at site-X in the cerebral cortex. This lesion is caused by the depletion of a particular neurotransmitter, Y-amine, which in turn is caused by a combination of autonomic nervous system overactivity (resulting from stress), a particularly rare dietary deficiency, and the endocrinological consequences of giving birth. Let us also suppose that Dr Neurone has obtained reasonable evidence that there is a typical constellation of symptoms that go with lesion-X, and that these symptoms include night-time wandering and the repetitious asking for help from anyone encountered. Perhaps Dr Neurone might also be able to demonstrate that these symptoms have a well-understood deteriorating course that can be completely reversed only by administering a corrective diet and a particular biochemical which is metabolised in the brain to restore the depleted Y-amine. Finally, Dr Neurone may have developed a pocket-sized nuclear magnetic resonance scanner which can reliably detect lesion-X and which has done so in the case of Mrs A. (Of course Szasz would argue that, in these circumstances, Mrs A would be suffering from a neurological rather than a psychiatric disorder,[20] but this has no implication for the present argument.) Would this strongest of possible cases justify the compulsory treatment of Mrs A?

That it is not sufficient to do so can be seen by considering two further hypothetical possibilities. Suppose that, having completed his research programme, Dr Neurone were to test Mrs A and find lesion-X to be absent? Would West therefore decide not to have her hospitalised? Alternatively, suppose that, during a routine laboratory demonstration for medical students, Dr Neurone was to discover that the Dean of his medical faculty (a female high-flyer just returned from maternity leave), despite showing no symptoms of the illness, was afflicted with lesion-X? In the face of the Dean's apparent rationality and understandable reluctance to enter a mental hospital would West have her compulsorily admitted for treatment?

Now, it is of course possible that West and his colleague Dr Neurone might want to argue that the Dean, despite apparent evidence to the contrary, does suffer from an illness, albeit of a sub-clinical variety. Medicine is replete with examples of illnesses which sometimes manifest themselves in a covert, sub-clinical fashion. Nevertheless, it is difficult to see why they would therefore want to deprive the Dean of her autonomy. It is quite conceivable that they would wish to persuade her of the virtues of receiving treatment for her condition, but what if she were to refuse (perhaps on the grounds that she was too busy and the illness was not troubling her)? In what way would this example be different from a situation in which the Dean has been afflicted by a nausea-causing virus but still insists on coming to work in order to catch up with her paperwork?

The point of these examples is to establish that the link between illness and compulsory treatment is more apparent than real. Even when illness is provable, it is not illness that justifies compulsory treatment. On the contrary, it is something about the behaviour of the ill person that does so. Curiously, the more the advocates of the medical model argue for the resemblance between mental and physical illness the more obvious this fact becomes.

IV

So it appears that, if he sticks to the illness criterion for depriving Mrs A of her liberty, West will become unstuck. He is therefore left with the option of finding something else that is different between the cases of Mrs A and Mr Z which will justify the compulsory treatment of the former and not the latter. What might this difference be?

An argument that West might make would be along the following lines: In contrast to Mr Z, Mrs A is not capable of making a rational choice about whether to consent to psychiatric treatment. Her behaviour is irrational or mad in the very real sense that it is not moved by reason. In parallel with West's previous argument with respect to illness, we can break down the hidden premises of this argument as follows: (2a) there is an objectively definable state which we can refer to as 'irrationality', (2b) that in at least some cases of irrationality it is justified to deprive the individual of his or her autonomy, and (2c) that unless someone is mad or irrational in this fashion it is not reasonable to deny them of their autonomy. Again, the burden of the argument is carried by (2b). In this case, however, any objection that East might make to (2b) seems less plausible. There does seem to be a logical connection between loss of rationality and loss of autonomy. The connection might most simply be put as follows: autonomy is not a static property of the individual but, rather, it has to be claimed. Persons who are unable to process information, weigh up evidence, and make choices accordingly cannot claim their autonomy no matter how much we might wish to award it to them. The point is that the concept of autonomy is inextricably linked to ideas about making rational judgements and rational judgements can only be made by persons who have adequately functioning cognitive mechanisms. It is therefore not surprising that some authors, for example Edwards[21] and Radden[22] have attempted to define madness or mental illness in terms of abnormal behaviour which evinces a lack of rational autonomy.

In this case, then, the validity of West's argument depends more on the convincingness of (2a). Now how could a state of irrationality be defined and identified? Radden[23] notes three philosophical traditions that have shaped present day accounts of irrationality: (a) irrational actions have sometimes been thought of as those actions which are socially or morally unacceptable; (b) irrational actions have been regarded as those actions which reduce the individual's expected utilities; and (c) irrational actions have sometimes been defined as those actions which are not based on good reasons. Each of these formulations of the distinction between rationality and irrationality present conceptual problems in their own right and these problems cannot be discussed in the present context for reasons of space. However, in parallel with my comments about the value of the illness criterion as a justification for compulsory treatment, I wish to show that, even if the conceptual problems surrounding definitions of irrationality could be solved, West would find any of the formulations of irrationality described by Radden problematic when it comes to distinguishing between the cases of Mrs A and Mr Z.

The problem with defining irrational acts as those acts which offend morally or socially is that it does not lead to an obvious justification of what West wants to do to Mrs A which is any different from the justification that East might offer with respect to the compulsory treatment of Mr Z. According to this criterion of irrationality, describing Mrs A as irrational amounts to nothing more than disapproving of what she does or what West suspects she is about to do. The dispute between West and East then becomes a dispute about what kinds of behaviour are socially or morally acceptable. Presumably, decisions about moral acceptability (even if the goal of an objective theory of ethics could be realised) must be imbedded in the social context of the person making the judgement. Western critics of Soviet psychiatry have generally overlooked this social context when leaping to condemn the psychiatric treatment of dissidents. Thus, as Lader points out,[24] Soviet conceptions of morality assume that the survival of the state (with the economic benefits it brings to Soviet citizens) is of paramount importance. Western critics of the Soviet regime have failed to make the distinction between two types of freedom – political freedom (most valued in the West) and economic freedom (most valued in the East). In condemning the Soviets it is as if they have performed a utilitarian computation while, in Soviet eyes at least, ignoring completely some of the most important utilities. There is nothing illogical about the Soviets regarding acts or beliefs which threaten the state as morally unacceptable or even bizarre.[25]

The second approach to defining irrational acts suggested by Radden is no more helpful to West's case. Given that the Soviets assign such high value to the survival of the State anyone who is threatening the State automatically reduces his or her own expected utility. Mr Z in particular does this in two ways. First, and importantly, he reduces the ability of the State to carry out its functions (to look after the interests of its citizens); in this respect there is a direct similarity between Mr Z's actions and those of Mrs A (which affect the cohesion of the family system). Second, and more trivially, Mr Z seriously incurs the wrath of his comrades much as Mrs A tries the patience of her neighbours.[26]

The third approach to defining irrational acts offers slightly more hope for West. In a version of this approach Davidson[27] has proposed three criteria that must be met by rational actions: that the reasons a person gives for the actions are in fact reasons for those actions; that the reasons do in fact cause the actions for which they are reasons; and that the reasons cause the actions in the right way. On this kind of analysis, irrationality might be demonstrated by a lack of consistency within a person's system of beliefs about how to achieve desired ends; a lack of consistency within the desires themselves; or a lack of consistency between a person's beliefs and desires on the one hand and the actions for which they are reasons on the other. Unfortunately, as Elster[28] points out, such consistency criteria provide only a 'thin' account of the distinction between rational and irrational conduct; a 'broader' account can be constructed by taking into consideration the nature of the beliefs and desires themselves (an issue which may be of some importance with respect to deluded patients). Irrational beliefs might thus be defined as those beliefs which are insufficiently grounded in the available evidence. Although it is much more difficult to construct criteria for irrational desires, Elster[29] has suggested that desires that are counter-adaptive or non-autonomous (for example, conformist desires) might qualify. Although there are many conceptual difficulties posed by this approach in general, it is clearly this kind of account that Edwards has in mind when he suggests that mental illness might be characterised by actions which fail to realise manifest goals; thinking that is illogical and replete with contradictions; beliefs that should be falsified by experience; the inability to give reasons for actions; unintelligible or nonsensical thinking; and a lack of impartiality or fair mindedness.[30]

Why, it might be asked, would someone persistently act irrationally (as defined by this approach)? One possibility is that such a person might act out of ignorance of information relevant to the particular circumstances in which he or she is placed. (Hence, there can be no such thing as uninformed consent.) Under certain situations it is entirely possible that a person may, by virtue of some condition, be so deprived of the information necessary to determine a rational course of action. A person in a coma, for example, cannot consent to treatment and consent must therefore be given by a proxy. (Technically, this kind of example would not be evidence of irrationality, at least in terms of a think theory of rationality, because there would be no inconsistency within beliefs, within desires, or between actions and the beliefs and desires which are reasons for those actions. Nonetheless, a person's behaviour might be thought of as non-rational under these circumstances because he or she is unable to make a rational choice.) More importantly for the present argument, a person may be irrational because, when provided with appropriate information, he or she is unable to make use of it as a consequence of suffering from some kind of mental or computational deficit; under these circumstances a person's behaviour might become very inconsistent and we might be inclined to describe such a person (loosely) as illogical.

This kind of approach to defining irrationality offers promise for two reasons. First, it fits in neatly with the logic linking irrationality with absence of autonomy previously outlined. Second, it avoids the pitfalls associated with defining irrationality (and hence madness) merely in terms of morally unacceptable behaviour. If West can demonstrate that Mrs A is irrational whereas Mr Z, is not, therefore, he has achieved his goal of finding a logical difference between the two cases.

This achievement can only be bought at a price, however. By defining irrationality in terms of a deficiency in reasoning, West has made the explanation, study and evaluation of irrationality part of the science of cognitive psychology. The assessment of irrationality would thus require the existence of a sophisticated understanding of human reasoning processes, and a method of detecting when those reasoning processes malfunction. The necessary tests would have to meet existing psychometric criteria of reliability (i.e. that they will achieve the same result no matter who administers them) and validity (i.e. that they measure what they purport to measure). In defence of his position, West might therefore introduce a second colleague, the world-renowned cognitive psychologist, Dr Ivan Cogito. Dr Cogito might report that he has, in fact, been working on an irrationality test[31] and that, when this test has been administered to Mrs A, it has indicated that she is unequivocally irrational. Of course, the widespread acceptance of a test of this sort would radically transform existing psychiatric practice; compulsory treatment orders are usually made on the basis of a medical practitioner's clinical judgement and formal tests are normally considered to be, at best, of only peripheral relevance. The amendment of existing mental health legislation would be necessary and the newly discovered tests would have to be recognised by courts and mental health tribunals. West and his colleagues might be willing to countenance such changes in order to draw a line between their practices and the practices of their Soviet colleagues. Nonetheless, there remain at least two practical reasons why their faith in Dr Cogito may prove premature.

First, existing psychological data on social and logical reasoning has been widely accepted as evidence that ordinary people often, perhaps usually, fail to reason in a rational and consistent fashion or make insufficient use of such evidence that may be relevant to their beliefs.[32] For example, social judgement has been found to be overly influenced by stereotypes and to be insensitive to statistical considerations such as the possible random covariation between events, the prior probabilities of events and the effect of sample sizes on the reliability of predictions.[33] Similarly, errors on inductive reasoning tasks are common because normal individuals (even those selected for high intelligence) fail to search for information which might disconfirm their hypotheses.[34] If irrationality of this sort is, as many psychologists believe, indeed the norm, the demonstration of some added degree of irrationality in mentally disturbed individuals might well prove difficult.

Second, and consistent with this argument, attempts to demonstrate irrationality in patients have often proved unconvincing. For example, although early workers argued that thought-disordered schizophrenic patients show deficits in logical reasoning, subsequent research has not born out this conclusion except for perhaps a minority of patients.[35] Patients suffering from hallucinations clearly meet the criteria for a broad account of irrationality as their beliefs about their perceptions are not well grounded in evidence.[36] However, it is not obvious that the paranoid patient necessarily meets either thin or broad criteria for irrationality (evidence that the delusions of such patients may have a rational basis has been already alluded to under II above). The problem of equating madness with irrationality is most clearly demonstrated with respect to severe depression, the (often life-threatening) emotional disorder which accounts for many compulsory psychiatric admissions in the West. In recent years there has in fact been a tendency to view the depressed patient as irrational because of his or her unduly pessimistic thoughts and beliefs; successful psychotherapy, on this view, is aimed at teaching the depressed patient to think more positively about life.[37] Unfortunately, there is no obvious reason to believe that pessimism alone indicates faulty reasoning, and the attribution of irrationality to depressed patients has been identified as a conceptual defect of the cognitive therapies.[38] Depressed patients often show precisely the kind of consistency in their reasoning about events that is required by the thin theory of rationality.[39] Moreover, one study found that depressed individuals were more accurate than normal controls on a task requiring the detection of covariation (i.e. they were less likely to believe that randomly associated events were causally connected), indicating that they were 'sadder but wiser'[40] and therefore more likely to meet the broad criteria of rationality than normal controls. The question of whether there can be such a thing as 'rational suicide' has proved particularly perplexing.[41] Finally, of course, there is the problem of the psychopath, who may be cold but who, more often than not, may appear completely rational.[42] In contrast to these types of cases, which often pose the most serious ethical problems for psychiatrists, it is perhaps only in cases of organic dementia or of extreme psychotic thought disorder that the capacity to demonstrate rational autonomy may be completely absent.

It must be emphasised once more that, according to the present argument, the use of irrationality to justify compulsory psychiatric treatment can only be made if a defect in the ability to reason can be demonstrated; this defect must be in principle demonstrable independently of the outcome of a particular judgement or series of decisions. Dr Cogito's tests, for example, must not fail to identify the individual who derives an apparently sensible conclusion on the basis of a series of bizarre associations. Nor must Dr Cogito's tests, through an insensitivity to the context in which people reach conclusions, identify persons as irrational simply because their actions seem unreasonable. It is just not good enough to say that mass-murderers must be mad, for example, without taking into account the manner in which they decide to commit their crimes. (What are we to make of nihilistic-anarchist terrorists, for example?) While it is not impossible for psychologists such as Dr Cogito to devise acceptable tests of irrationality, the likelihood that even the most severely disturbed psychiatric patients will be found irrational seems remote.

V

At least one line of argument remains open to West. He can abandon all pretence that the decision to hospitalise Mrs A is a clinical judgement pure and simple based on an assessment of Mrs A's mental illness or (alternatively) her degree of rationality. He may simply concede that, after all, he, or at least society in general (on whose behalf he acts as an agent) disapproves of some forms of behaviour because such behaviour seems morally wrong, and that his job is that of a benign policeman – to arrest and contain those who persistently evince such behaviour. The role of the psychiatrist in containing the behaviour of the psychopath clearly fits this model. Indeed, unless irrationality can be demonstrated, it would seem that this may be the only role left open to the psychiatrist.

If this argument is correct, two consequences follow. First, West and East are in the same boat, whether they like it or not, and the dispute about the treatment of Mrs A and Mr Z amounts to no more than an ideological difference. This does not mean that West's case against East must fail but it does mean that it can only be based on the ethical analysis of individual cases and of the political regimes in which they occur.

The second consequence has already been alluded to and concerns West's professional role. Like East, he is acting as a kind of policeman. The judgements that he makes about the treatment of his patients, despite appearances to the contrary, have little to do with medicine but have everything to do with the moral evaluation of conduct. But West has no more expertise in this area than any of the rest of us. He is, or at least should be, functioning as our spokesman.

VI

In the end, then, it would seem that it is not possible to legitimately deprive someone of their autonomy merely because they are ill. People who are irrational, however, cannot be deprived of their autonomy because they are unable to claim it in the first place. A convincing case for compulsory psychiatric treatment can therefore be made in those cases in which the individual is demonstrably irrational, so long as irrationality is defined in a certain way. In particular, for the argument to work the criterion employed for irrationality must make reference to cognitive functioning and not to outcomes or expected utilities of actions. This may be possible in certain cases of extreme psychosis or in the case of the organic dementias, but it is not clear that it is possible in the case of one of the most common reasons for compulsory treatment – severe depression. Moreover, proponents of the irrationality criterion have yet to find ways of defining irrationality in a manner that excludes the everyday defects of reasoning demonstrated by cognitive psychologists or of assessing irrationality in a manner which would satisfy the psychometricians's criteria for reliability or validity.

In the absence of demonstrable irrationality, the psychiatrist can only fall back on moral disapproval of the actions of the person who is to be compelled into receiving treatment. In this role it is simply a fact that the psychiatrist (be he Western or Soviet) is functioning as an agent of the state.

Notes

1. The case of Mrs A is taken from a talk on psychiatric ethics given at University College Cardiff by Dr Sidney Bloch, then consultant psychotherapist at the Warneford Hospital, Oxford. I have chosen to use this case to illustrate my argument because Dr Bloch, making a similar comparison to the one made here, reached somewhat different conclusions than myself. In fact, most examples of involuntary

hospitalisation that arise in modern psychiatric practice would do equally well.

2. There can be no doubt that this sort of thing does happen in the Soviet Union. See M. Lader, *Psychiatry on Trial* (Harmondsworth: Penguin, 1977) and S. Bloch 'The Political Misuse of Psychiatry in the Soviet Union', in S. Bloch and P. Chodoff (eds), *Psychiatric Ethics* (Oxford: Oxford University Press, 1981).
3. See M. Lader, ibid., and S. Bloch, ibid. See also W. Reich, 'Psychiatric diagnosis as an ethical problem', in Bloch and Chodoff, ibid.
4. S. Bloch, 'Political Misuse'.
5. T. Szasz, *The Myth of Mental Illness: Foundations of a Theory of Personal Conduct* (New York: Hoeber-Harper, 1961).
6. T. Scheff, *Being Mentally Ill: A Sociological Theory* (Chicago: Aldine, 1966).
7. See, for example, A. Bandura, *Principles of Behaviour Modification* (Englewood Cliffs: Prentice Hall, 1969); and L. Ullmann and L. Krasner, *A Psychological Approach to Abnormal Behaviour* (New York: Appleton-Century-Crofts, 1975).
8. See J. K. Wing *Reasoning About Madness* (Oxford: Oxford University Press, 1978).
9. If this is not the aim of placing mental disorder with the scope of the concept of 'illness' it is difficult to see what the argument is about. Otherwise we would be justified in asking, 'Why should it matter whether schizophrenia is an illness?' People sometimes talk of our 'sick' society but no one worries whether this is the misuse of a medical concept.
10. I find these arguments unconvincing, not least on empirical grounds. See R. P. Bentall, 'The Scientific Validity of the Schizophrenia Diagnosis: A Critical Evaluation', in N. Eisenberg and D. Glasgow (eds), *Current Issues in Clinical Psychology* (Aldershot: Gower, 1986) and R. P. Bentall, H. F. Jackson and D. Pilgrim, 'On abandoning the concept of schizophrenia: Some implications of validity arguments for psychological research into psychotic phenomena', *British Journal of Clinical Psychology* (in press).
11. Chronic amphetamine abuse often leads to paranoid symptoms. See B. Angrist and S. Gershon, 'The Phenomenology of Experimentally Induced Amphetamine Psychosis: Preliminary Observations', *Biological Psychiatry*, vol. 2, pp. 95–107.
12. See N. C. Andreasen, *The Broken Brain* (New York: Harper and Row, 1984). Dr Andreasen is a lucid advocate of the biological approach.
13. R. D. Laing, *The Divided Self* (London: Tavistock, 1962); and *The Politics of Experience* (London: Tavistock, 1967).
14. See, for example, M. Roth and J. Kroll, *The Reality of Mental Illness*

(Cambridge: Cambridge University Press, 1986) for a rejection of Laing's position from the standpoint of biological psychiatry. See D. Bannister, 'The psychotic disguise', in W. Dryden (ed.), *Therapist's Dilemmas* (London: Croom-Helm, 1987) for a psycholgical account of delusions.

15. R. D. Laing and A. Eesterson, *Sanity, Madness and the Family* (Harmondsworth: Penguin, 1970).
16. See M. Roth and J. Kroll, *The Reality of Mental Illness.*
17. See in particular the work of the Milan school of family therapy and their followers, for example: M. Selvini Palazzoli and G. Prata, 'A New Method for Therapy and Research in the Treatment of Schizophrenic Families', in H. Stierlin, L. C. Wynne and M. Wirching (eds), *Psychosocial Interventions in Schizophrenia* (Berlin: Springer-Verlag, 1983); and E. Jones, 'Brief systemic work in psychiatric settings where a family member has been diagnosed as schizophrenic', *Journal of Family Therapy* (1987) vol. 9, pp. 3–25. For a rather different perspective on the family therapy of psychotic individuals see J. Leff, L. Kuipers, R. Berkowitz, R. Eberlein-Vries and D. Sturgeon, 'A controlled trial of social intervention in the families of schizophrenic patients', *British Journal of Psychiatry* (1982) vol. 141, pp. 121–34.
18. See, for example, R. H. Forgus and A. S. DeWolfe, 'Coding of cognitive input in delusional patients', *Journal of Abnormal Psychology* (1974) vol. 83, pp. 278–84; W. G. Johnson, J. M. Ross and M. Mastria, 'Delusional behaviour: An attributional analysis of development and modification', *Journal of Abnormal Psychology* (1977) vol. 86, pp. 421–26; and D. R. Hemsley and P. A. Garety, 'The formation and maintenance of delusions: A Bayesian analysis', *British Journal of Psychiatry* (1986) vol. 149, pp. 51–6.
19. See F. N. Watts, E. G. Powell and S. V. Austin, 'The modification of abnormal beliefs', *British Journal of Medical Psychology*, (1973) vol. 46 pp. 359–63; and L. M. Hartman and F. E. Cashmana, 'Cognitive-behavioural and psycopharmacological treatment of delusional symptoms', *Behavioural Psychotherapy* (1983) vol. 11, pp. 50–61.
20. Szasz, *The Myth of Mental Illness.*
21. See R. B. Edwards, 'Mental health as rational autonomy', *International Journal of Medicine and Philosophy* (1961) vol. 6, pp. 309–22.
22. J. Radden, *Madness and Reason* (London: George Allen and Unwin, 1985).
23. Ibid.
24. Lader, *Psychiatry on Trial.*
25. Of course, West might want to argue that the Soviet political regime is in fact morally wrong in certain ways. However, this will not allow him to find a logical difference between the cases of Mrs A and Mr Z.

26. Utilitarian considerations of this sort are enshrined in mental health legislation in Britain and the United States. For example, legislation in Britain states that a disorder of mind might warrant detention for treatment if treatment is necessary in the interest of the patient's health or safety or for the protection of others. See L. McGarry and P. Chodoff, 'The ethics of involuntary hospitalisation', in S. Bloch and P. Chodoff (eds), *Psychiatric Ethics*.
27. D. Davidson, *Essays on Actions and Events* (Oxford: Oxford University Press, 1980).
28. J. Elster, *Sour Grapes: Studies on the Subversion of Rationality* (Cambridge: Cambridge University Press, 1983).
29. Ibid.
30. Edwards, 'Mental health as rational autonomy'.
31. For discussion of the relative strengths and weaknesses of some simple possible tests of rationality, see L. H. Roth, A. Meisel and C. W. Lidz, 'Tests of competency to consent to treatment', *American Journal of Psychiatry* (1977) vol. 134, pp. 279–84.
32. See, for example, H. R. Arkes and K. R. Hammond (eds), *Judgement and Decision Making: An Interdisciplinary Reader* (Cambridge: Cambridge University Press, 1986); L. J. Cohen, 'Can human irrationality be experimentally demonstrated', *The Behavioural and Brain Sciences* (1981) vol. 4, pp. 317–31; and E. Nisbett and L. Ross, *Human Inference: Strategies and Shortcomings of Human Judgement* (Englewood Cliffs: Prentice-Hall, 1980).
33. See R. Nisbett and L. Ross, ibid.
34. See, for example, K. J. Gilhooly, *Thinking: Directed, Undirected and Creative* (London: Academic Press, 1982).
35. The idea that schizophrenics are illogical is usually attributed to E. Von Domarus (1944). The specific laws of logic in schizophrenia are set out in J. S. Kasanin (ed.), *Language and Thought in Schizophrenia* (Berkeley: University of California Press). Although many cognitive deficits have subsequently been attributed to schizophrenics, the view that they suffer from a specific logical deficit has not been born out by subsequent research, see L. J. Chapman and J. P. Chapman, *Disordered Thought in Schizophrenia* (Englewood Cliffs: Prentice-Hall, 1973); and J. M. Neale and T. Oltmanns, *Schizophrenia* (New York: Wiley, 1980).
36. For evidence that hallucinations should be thought of as errors of judgement, see R. P. Bentall and P. D. Slade, 'Reality testing and auditory hallucinations: A signal detection analysis', *British Journal of Clinical Psychology* (1985) vol. 24, pp. 159–69.
37. This has become perhaps the dominant psychological theory of depression. See A. Beck, *Cognitive Therapy and the Emotional Disorders* (New York: International Universities Press, 1976); and J. M. G.

Williams, *The Psychological Treatment of Depression* (London: Croom Helm, 1984).

38. M. J. Mahoney, *Cognition and Behaviour Modification* (New York: Ballinger, 1974).
39. See Beck, *Cognitive Therapy*.
40. C. B. Alloy and L. Y. Abramson, 'Judgement of contingency in depressed and non-depressed students: Sadder but wiser', *Journal of Experimental Psychology: General*, (1979) vol. 108, pp. 441–85.
41. See T. Szasz, 'The ethics of suicide', *The Antioch Review* (1971) vol. 31, pp. 7–17; and D. Heyd and S. Bloch, 'The ethics of suicide', in S. Bloch and P. Chodoff (eds), *Psychiatric Ethics*.
42. See R. D. Hare and D. Schalling (eds), *Psychopathic Behaviour Approaches to Research* (New York: Wiley, 1978).

Index